1-05

Reproductive Technology

Reproductive Technology

Other books in the At Issue series:

Reproductive Technology

Cindy Mur, *Book Editor*

Bruce Glassman, *Vice President*
Bonnie Szumski, *Publisher*
Helen Cothran, *Managing Editor*

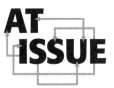 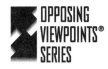

GREENHAVEN PRESS
An imprint of Thomson Gale, a part of The Thomson Corporation

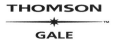
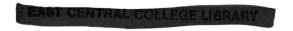

THOMSON
GALE

Detroit • New York • San Francisco • San Diego • New Haven, Conn.
Waterville, Maine • London • Munich

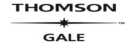

For more information, contact
Greenhaven Press
27500 Drake Rd.
Farmington Hills, MI 48331-3535
Or you can visit our Internet site at http://www.gale.com

LIBRARY OF CONGRESS CATALOGING-IN-PUBLICATION DATA

Reproductive technology / Cindy Mur, book editor.
    p. cm. — (At issue)
  Includes bibliographical references and index.
  ISBN 0-7377-2412-9 (lib. : alk. paper) — ISBN 0-7377-2413-7 (pbk. : alk. paper)
    1. Human reproductive technology. 2. Human reproductive technology—
  Moral and ethical aspects. I. Mur, Cindy. II. At issue (San Diego, Calif.)
  RG133.5.R458 2005
  176—dc22   2004046079

Contents

Introduction

When Louise Brown was born in 1978 in England, she became the world's first baby to be born as a result of a procedure called in vitro fertilization (IVF). Since that time, IVF has grown into a multimillion dollar industry. More than 114,000 babies have been born as a result of this technology in the United States, bringing joy to thousands of couples. Of those who seek medical attention for infertility, 5 percent utilize in vitro fertilization.

The IVF process begins in a laboratory. A technician removes and then fertilizes several oocytes—immature egg cells—with sperm in a petri dish to create fertilized eggs. Some of these are selected for transfer to the mother's uterus a few days later.

The IVF procedure has some inherent problems. First, not every implantation results in the birth of a baby. Successful birthrates vary by clinic but average about 29.4 percent per egg retrieval, according to the American Society for Reproductive Medicine (ASRM). Each egg retrieval involves the removal of at least three and as many as a fifteen eggs from the woman for fertilization. Usually, only two to four embryos are implanted at one time. Since not every implantation results in pregnancy, multiple implantations may be necessary to achieve childbirth. Second, the process can be physically painful. The woman must inject herself with hormones every day for seven to ten days to stimulate egg production, and she may have to have progesterone shots or suppositories to facilitate implantation and pregnancy. An additional obstacle is that the procedure is expensive, costing an average of $12,400 in the United States for each egg retrieval, according to ASRM. Very few insurance plans cover this expense—and only a few states mandate that insurance companies provide IVF coverage.

One of the most serious consequences of the IVF procedure is the creation of surplus frozen embryos. According to Nicholas Wade, science editor for the *New York Times*, "Because of the expense and inconvenience of extracting an egg for in vitro fertilization, couples prefer to extract a large number of eggs at once so that others will be on hand if the first implantation fails."

Columnist Jeremy Manier of the *Chicago Tribune* explains further: "Leftover embryos are a common result of in-vitro fertilization . . . most clinics will create a dozen or more embryos during a given round of IVF treatment, but implant only the two or three embryos that grow best or seem most likely to survive in the womb."

The result of this practice is that almost four hundred thousand frozen human embryos are currently preserved in fertility clinics in the United States, according to a survey published in 2003 by the Society for Assisted Reproductive Technology. Approximately 87 percent of these embryos are being kept for possible future use by the parents, the survey found.

Once a couple has decided they will not implant their remaining embryos, they have several options: The embryos can be donated for research, donated for adoption, or destroyed. The decision about what to do with surplus frozen embryos raises many ethical issues. The central debate, however, is whether humanity has the right to manipulate or destroy life.

Embryo use in research

Those who donate their frozen embryos for research do so because they believe that others can be helped by it. According to health columnist Kevin Lamb, "The clear scientific consensus is that [embryos] also offer the best potential for saving people from Alzheimer's disease and other debilitating brain disorders, diabetes and spinal-cord injuries, among many afflictions." Embryos are valuable in research because they contain stem cells—undifferentiated cells that can develop into any parts of the body. Those cells can be used to rejuvenate or replace dying or diseased tissue and thus may eventually be useful in combating illnesses like Parkinson's disease that attack nerve or brain tissue. In the future, doctors may be able to extract tissue from a patient, create a cloned embryo, and use that embryo's stem cell tissue to create needed organs the recipient's body will not reject. This could be a lifesaving procedure for the thousands of patients on donor waiting lists.

Despite its potential to save lives, opponents of embryo research think using a frozen embryo for research purposes is wrong. They believe embryos are potential lives and that it is therefore inhuman to experiment on them. The Center for Bioethics and Human Dignity likens embryo research to the medical experiments performed on prisoners at Auschwitz, a

German concentration camp during World War II. Opponents also point out that researchers can use adult stem cells in their studies rather than needlessly destroying embryos.

Embryo adoption

Many people opposed to embryo stem cell research believe that donating frozen embryos for adoption by another couple is the best solution to the problem of excess frozen embryos. A potential life is not lost and an infertile couple receives the possibility of having a child. As Father Joseph Howard states in the journal *Human Life Review*, "There is an ethical obligation to do what one can to save a life." In 2002 the federal government supported embryo adoption by creating a $1 million program to promote it.

Embryo adoption has been labeled a godsend by the infertile couples who who have chosen it. A woman who receives a donated embryo has the chance to experience childbirth, and the couple may begin caring for the child almost from conception. In addition, the cost for the adopting couple is much less prohibitive than with traditional in vitro methods because they do not have the expense of fertility shots or of harvesting the eggs—they must only pay for implantation. Some couples have even claimed a federal adoption tax credit.

However, some people argue against the adoption of embryos. They believe that allowing adoption only legitimizes the practice of creating more embryos than needed. Instead, they think that no extra embryos should be produced. Some critics believe that creating extra embryos and not using them is the same as abandoning children.

Many religious leaders are also critical of embryo adoption. William Smith, a monsignor and professor of moral theology at St. Joseph's Seminary in New York City, believes that adopting an embryo "amounts to a form of high-tech surrogate motherhood, which distorts natural sexual and family relations," as reported by Brian Caulfield in *Human Life Review.* Smith states that, while those who wish to adopt embryos have good intentions, the act violates the "underlying principles of the procreative act and the nature of marriage." Other religious leaders, such as Bishop Elio Sgreccia of the Pontifical Academy for Life, are hesitant to counsel women to choose embryo adoption because they believe that the freezing and thawing process may cause many embryos to suffer genetic damage.

The legal status of embryos is another important issue in embryo adoption. The main debate is whether frozen embryos should be considered property or people with rights. Right-to-life organizations argue that embryos should be afforded the same rights as any person. As columnist Jeremy Manier reports, some of these organizations believe that people who wish to adopt an embryo should submit to the same background checks and home visits required for traditional adoptions. However, embryo adoption is not necessarily the same as adopting a child because the adopting mother carries and gives birth to the child. As legal expert Lori Andrews points out, "One reason the adoption model would be wrong for embryo donation is that the adoption process is supposed to screen would-be parents to confirm they are committed to raising a child. Embryo donation is different because most state laws presume that a woman who carries a child to birth has earned the right to be a parent."

If background checks for adopting parents became a requirement, not only might the legal status of the embryo change, but the costs for the adopting parents would increase significantly.

Regardless of the moral and legal arguments, for many parents the decision to place an embryo up for adoption is a personal, emotional one. In fact, most couples feel uncomfortable donating their surplus frozen embryos and dislike the idea of giving their potential offspring to a stranger. According to a 2001 study of patients at Northwestern Memorial Hospital in Chicago, only 13 percent of couples preferred donating their extra embryos for adoption. Almost one-third preferred having them destroyed.

Embryo destruction

Ultimately, some couples decide the best course of action is to dispose of their surplus embryos. Embryos are usually destroyed by being thawed and allowed to resume their cell division until they can no longer continue to grow outside of a uterus because there is no nourishment, at which point they die. In some instances, they are plunged in a hot solution—termed "rapid thaw." In both instances, the embryos are then discarded as biological waste. Some women have the embryos implanted during a time of the month when pregnancy is unlikely so that they can die "naturally." Some couples are unfazed by the disposal of their embryos. Others bury them, or they watch when the embryos are disposed of by the fertility clinic. Many women, like Martha Panak of Richmond, Virginia, feel an emotion that lies between the detachment one feels toward an object and the love one has for a child. She has four frozen embryos and commented in a *Redbook* article that "they're more than just a bunch of cells . . . I don't view them in the same way as my children . . . [but] we have an emotional attachment to them."

Religious laws concerning embryo destruction vary. Jewish law prohibits the destruction of a fetus, but does not prohibit disposing of an embryo outside the womb. The Catholic Church, however, believes that life begins at conception—defined by the church as the point at which the egg is fertilized by the sperm. Therefore, the church likens the destruction of an embryo to abortion. Evangelical Christian groups agree. As JoAnn Davidson of the Christian Adoption and Family Services states, embryos "are life from the moment of conception. . . . There's only that one unique moment when the sperm and egg come together, and everything else is just stages of development."

Embryos in storage

As outlined above, both religious and personal beliefs factor into a couple's decision about what to do with their surplus frozen embryos. Undeniably, the choice is a difficult one, and so hundreds of thousands of embryos are left in storage in fertility clinics. Robert J. Stillman, medical director of Shady Grove Reproductive Science Center in Washington, D.C., explains in a *Redbook* interview the difficult choice couples with frozen embryos face: "They just can't bear to give their 'child' to research, and they don't want it disposed of, and they certainly don't want it running around in somebody else's house. . . . So they make a non-decision."

In some cases, couples abandon their embryos by no longer paying for their storage fees. In 1996 British authorities destroyed almost three thousand abandoned frozen embryos, which led to a law in the United Kingdom limiting storage time for embryos to five years. As of May 2003, there were fifty-two thousand frozen embryos in the United Kingdom. The United States allows unlimited storage time, which helps explain why there are four hundred thousand frozen embryos in storage. To handle the burden, facilities that serve solely as storage for frozen embryos have opened.

The debates over when life begins and over whether it is ever acceptable to manipulate or even destroy potential life reflect the many issues that are at stake in the field of reproductive technology. The authors in *At Issue: Reproductive Technology* address the ethical questions that arise with the continuing scientific discovery in the field of reproduction.

1

In Vitro Fertilization Increases the Likelihood of Multiple and Premature Births

Maggie Jones

Maggie Jones is a Los Angeles–based freelance journalist who writes about social, health, and women's issues. Her articles have appeared in the New York Times Magazine, *the* Washington Post, Parenting, *and other publications.*

The incidence of multiple births has increased dramatically in the last two decades, primarily because of reproductive technologies like in vitro fertilization (IVF). With IVF, women are usually implanted with several embryos in order to increase their chance of conception. As a result, many more women give birth to twins or triplets. Women pregnant with more than one baby usually give birth prematurely—in many cases at twenty-eight weeks or earlier. These premature babies are vulnerable to physical ailments such as lung problems or learning disabilities. Some premature babies weigh about a pound and may not live more than a few days. The problem originates with fertility clinics that compete for business by advertising pregnancy success rates—the greater the number of embryos implanted, the better their chance for success. Women who desperately want to become pregnant will risk multiple births.

L ike so many other thirtysomething women, Nicki Azoff turned to a fertility clinic to get pregnant. Six months later, her twins joined the growing ranks of preemies clinging to life at a Boston hospital.

> *First, you notice the babies. Some so tiny, each fits into the palm of a doctor's hand and weighs no more than a few apples.*

First, you notice the babies. Some so tiny, each fits into the palm of a doctor's hand and weighs no more than a few apples. Their skin is paper-thin. Their limbs are spindly twigs. Then you notice something else about the Neonatal Intensive Care Unit (NICU) at Beth Israel Deaconess Medical Center: Twins and triplets are everywhere. Multiples can sometimes account for more than half of the unit's babies. Doctors and nurses call one area of this hospital unit "Twin Alley."

Multiple birth trends

In the last two decades, the rate of triplets and higher-order multiple births has rocketed a staggering 400 percent, leading to a dramatic upsurge in the number of premature babies. It's the result of a booming fertility industry, aided by women who wait longer to give birth—particularly in this state. In 1996, Massachusetts became the first state in which more babies were born to women 30 and older than to women under 30, and the trend has only escalated since. "We were narrowing the problems of prematurity in Massachusetts," says Dr. DeWayne Pursley, head of Beth Israel's NICU. "Then assisted reproductive technology came around." While a normal pregnancy lasts 37 to 42 weeks, twins are born on average at 35 weeks, triplets at 33 weeks, and quadruplets at 30 weeks. Most of these babies will be healthy. But as fertility clinics spin out more multiples, many of those twins, triplets, and quadruplets will be born extremely premature—at 28 weeks or less—when infants are most vulnerable to lung problems, brain hemorrhages, learning disabilities, and cerebral palsy.

"Couples see twins as two for the price of one," says Dr. Richard Reindollar, a reproductive endocrinologist at the fertility clinic Boston IVF. "It's true the majority will do fine. Still, I know about 6 percent of twins die in the second trimester." Another 6 percent will spend three to five days in the NICU. And 12 percent will be in the unit for a few weeks or more, sometimes living in incubators that serve as high-tech wombs. Connected to monitors and ventilators that beep and buzz and ring, the incubators keep babies alive, Reindollar says, until they can survive in the outside world.

"Twins," he says, "are not a success."

Getting pregnant through in vitro fertilization

Nicki Azoff and her husband, Peter, had wanted a baby since they married in 1992. Even their jobs were child-oriented: Peter was a school furniture sales rep; Nicki, a pediatric occupational therapist. Doctors couldn't explain the Natick [Massachusetts] couple's infertility, so over two years they did four in vitro fertilization (IVF) procedures. Morning and night, Nicki injected her thighs with fertility hormones. She had ultrasounds and blood tests every few days. Then, during each IVF procedure, doctors anesthetized her and pierced her ovarian follicles with a needle to retrieve the eggs. In the lab, the eggs were fertilized with Peter's sperm and, a few days later, the resulting embryos were transferred to Nicki's uterus.

But after three rounds of IVF, Nicki was 32, still not pregnant, and increasingly desperate. On her fourth try, none of the embryos looked particularly healthy, so Nicki, Peter, and their doctor agreed to transfer five embryos into Nicki's uterus instead of three or four.

For all her infertility heartaches, Nicki was fortunate in one way: She lived in Massachusetts, probably the most infertile-friendly state in the country. The largest fertility center in the United States is Boston IVF, which has three clinics in Greater Boston and performs an extraordinary 3,000 IVF procedures each year at a typical cost of about $10,000 per round. The state also ranks third overall for most fertility procedures performed, behind only California and New York. And when it comes to insurance coverage, it doesn't get much better than Massachusetts, which is one of only four states that mandates comprehensive coverage for IVF.

Such benefits were nonexistent a generation ago when most babies were born to women in their twenties—the peak of fertility. But by 1996 that trend had changed in Massachusetts, probably because of the number of highly educated, career-focused women who delay childbearing until their jobs and their personal lives are settled.

Older motherhood undoubtedly has plenty of advantages. Women over 30 are less likely to smoke. They tend to be more financially stable and emotionally mature than their younger counterparts. But there are two potential downsides to waiting: Infertility. And premature babies.

A triple pregnancy

During an ultrasound following Nicki's fourth IVF, her doctor beamed. There are three heartbeats, he announced. Triplets. Lying on the examining table, Nicki looked at Peter with worry. They had longed for a baby for years. But they'd never imagined three. The expenses—and the stress—would be enormous. Mostly, though, Peter questioned whether Nicki, just 5 feet tall and thin, could carry three babies to term. "Both of our hearts just sank," Nicki says.

Women faced with carrying triplets and quadruplets often undergo a procedure called multifetal reduction—the termination of one or more embryos or fetuses during the first trimester to improve the odds that the others will be born healthy. "The parents have heard the statistics about multiples resulting from fertility treatments," says Dr. Linda Heffner, head of maternal-fetal medicine at Brigham and Women's Hospital. "But they never expected they were going to have triplets. And no one's talked to them about the implications." Of the 100 or so patients who consult with Heffner and her partner annually, about half choose to reduce their pregnancies to twins.

Like many women in her situation, Nicki couldn't bear the thought of fetal reduction. By the eighth week of her pregnancy, she didn't have to. During a followup ultrasound, she learned one of the embryos had died. Nicki wasn't sure how to feel: After years of trying to get pregnant, she'd lost an embryo. But she knew the others would have a better shot now. In the coming months, she would learn that the twins were boys. And as her belly grew, Nicki relished the thought of being their mother.

The source of the problem

When Beth Israel's NICU opened [in 1992], the staff underestimated the number of babies they would see each month. "We were counting expectant mothers," says Dr. Pursley, "when we should have been counting fetuses." As nurses wheeled more incubators with twins and triplets into the unit, some doctors grew increasingly alarmed. Among them was Dr. Douglas K. Richardson, one of the unit's seven highly respected neonatologists. (He was interviewed by *Boston* magazine in July [2003], a month before he died in a bicycling accident.) "There's no interaction between fertility clinics and NICUs," Richardson complained. "From the perspective of most fertility doctors, it's irrelevant if one out of six mothers ends up with babies in the NICU. Their thinking is: Women want to be pregnant, and we get them pregnant. The idea that these pregnancies run up huge NICU bills and cause untold suffering doesn't seem relevant to them."

The problem stems in part from the competitive nature of the fertility industry. Clinics advertise their success rates, and women flock to the ones that boast the best odds. "And how do you guarantee the highest rates of success?" Richardson said. "Implant more embryos."

> *Parents have heard the statistics about multiples resulting from fertility treatments. . . . But they never expected they were going to have triplets.*

Doctors, bioethicists, and fertility organizations have been debating whether federal regulations are needed to restrict the number of embryos doctors can transfer during in vitro procedures. Laws in Sweden, England, and some other countries generally restrict doctors from implanting more than one or two embryos. Few expect such regulations in the United States. Three years ago, the American Society for Reproductive Medicine, the nation's largest organization of fertility doctors, issued guidelines—which are completely voluntary—suggesting doctors implant no more than three embryos in any woman under 35. And even as improved lab techniques offer better ways for doctors to select the best (and fewest) embryos to implant, the multiple rate remains startlingly high. While only 1.2 percent of natural pregnancies result in twins, the overall likelihood that women under 35 pregnant through IVF will deliver multiples is an incredible 40 percent nationwide—and only slightly lower in Massachusetts.

The IVF multiple rates at most Boston clinics are 30 to 35 percent. And as long as fertility doctors are rewarded for their high pregnancy rates and women are willing to gamble on multiples, many doctors don't expect those numbers to substantially decrease soon. "Women have gone through so much and invested so much that they'll take risks," said Richardson. "The women want it, and the doctors don't want to deny it."

Two premature births

One morning during a staff meeting at work, Nicki felt waves of sharp pain in her back. By 11 P.M., she was admitted to Beth Israel's Labor and Delivery Unit. Her water had broken; the contractions, which Nicki would later learn may have been brought on by an infection in her uterus, were three minutes apart. She was barely six months pregnant.

Nicki knew that even an additional day in the womb could mean the difference between her babies living and dying. "I am not having these babies now," she told her obstetrician, with Peter by her side. But doctors had no way to stop Nicki's premature labor without putting the fetuses at risk. Four hours later, the babies were on their way.

Max came out first. Then Seth was born, his thin skin badly bruised by the trauma of the delivery. Max weighed 1 pound, 9 ounces, and Seth, 3 ounces less. Neither was longer than 12 inches. Their purple, wrinkled skin hung from their scrawny limbs like an old man's. Their eyes were fused shut. They looked more like fetuses than newborns. Under heat lamps, two teams of NICU doctors, nurses, and respiratory therapists worked at a furious pace, assessing each baby for breathing and heart rates. Seth and Max weren't crying or screaming, declaring themselves alive the way full-term babies do. They were barely breathing. Nicki prayed for at least one to live.

In minutes, doctors threaded spaghetti-like breathing tubes into the babies' throats and whisked them down the hall in incubators. Seth and Max were gone before Nicki or Peter had been able to hold or even touch them.

Left in the delivery room with Peter and a nurse, Nicki started crying. "I want a room anywhere but the maternity wing," she told the nurse. Believing that the babies she'd tried to conceive for more than two years were about to die, she didn't want to spend her recovery watching healthy, plump newborns head home with their glowing parents.

Twenty-five years ago, Max and Seth would have had little chance of surviving. But in recent decades, neonatology's leaps have been among the most impressive in medicine. With the invention of mechanical ventilators in the late 1960s, babies that had been in the womb for only 34 weeks were routinely saved. In the next two decades, improved intravenous nutrition and more sophisticated ventilators rescued babies as young as 26 weeks. And by the late 1980s, almost 100 percent of 34-weekers and 90 percent of babies born after pregnancies of 27 to 31 weeks were surviving. More recently, synthetic surfactant, the substance that helps [keep] babies' lungs from collapsing, has helped push survival rates for 24-weekers like Max and Seth from 10 percent to 50 percent.

But for all its high-tech gadgetry, neonatology remains a game of chance. With the smallest babies, doctors make educated guesses about their long-term outcomes. "We do our best to make the right decisions," Beth Israel's Dr. DeWayne Pursley says. "But in one of out of four scenarios, you don't know what's going to happen."

Working to save the babies

Within minutes of the babies' arrival in the NICU, all the technology and know-how of the past decades came together to try to save them. Doctors and nurses hooked up Max and Seth to ventilators and attached a mass of wires to their feet, chests, and stomachs. The babies were fed through intravenous lines in their belly buttons. Overhead, monitors flashed their heart rates and blood pressure. Still, Seth's lungs were so underdeveloped that even the most gentle ventilator setting was too harsh: The air pressure that helped inflate Seth's lungs also blew holes in his lungs.

Seth, the smaller of the babies, had been alive for 10 hours when the NICU staff called Nicki and Peter to his bedside. Though they had expected bad news, the couple held out hope. But neonatologist Dr. Jim Gray explained that Seth's lungs were irreparably damaged. He then gently offered Nicki and Peter a choice: Seth could die while hooked up to the ventilator, or he could die in his parents' arms. If only for a short while, Nicki and Peter wanted to parent their infant without the wires and machines.

As the respiratory therapist shut off the ventilator, Gray pulled the tube out of Seth's trachea. Then, one of the nurses wrapped Seth in a blanket and brought him to a small room in the NICU usually used for mothers to pump breast milk for their newborns. Still dressed in her hospital gown, Nicki was holding Seth in her arms when he died 20 minutes later.

Shortly after Seth's death, a nurse gave Nicki and Peter a small silk box from the NICU social workers and the rest of the staff. Inside were photos of Seth, his baby cap, a poem, a note from the staff, and a lock of Seth's hair—the mementos of his brief life.

> *What had begun as a triplet pregnancy was now reduced to one baby with a precarious hold on life.*

What had begun as a triplet pregnancy was now reduced to one baby with a precarious hold on life. In his first week of life, Max had a 40 percent chance of dying from ripped lung sacs, infections, or other complications. During morning rounds the day after Seth's death, Richardson looked at Max in his incubator. "The parents' hopes are in one remaining fragile basket," he said. But Nicki and Peter clung to the flip side of the statistics: If Max could make it through those first weeks, he would have a 50 percent chance of growing up as a kid with no greater handicap than a pair of glasses or a slow finish in school relay races.

"I'm sorry, handsome," murmured nurse Linda Mahoney, turning Max on his side and rearranging the sheepskin he slept on. "I know you hate this." Max twisted his face and trembled at Mahoney's touch. Even opening the incubator porthole—which Mahoney did several times a day to change Max's doll-sized diapers, check his temperature, and occasionally prick his heel for a blood test—caused his temperature to drop. After shutting the incubator, Mahoney turned to a computer to update Max's chart. A few moments later, his eyes still closed, Max stretched out his hand, like a blind man searching for a bearing. But there was nothing—no womb, no mother. Just air.

Sometimes Nicki allowed herself to think about how it was supposed to be. If the twins had held on, if they had made it to

38 or 40 weeks instead of 24, she would have spent her mornings in her three-bedroom suburban house. She'd wake up when her sons woke up. She'd breast-feed them and dress them in cotton rompers, socks, and caps. She'd put them in strollers and take them to the neighborhood park.

Struggling to go home

Instead, Nicki spent every day in an intensive care unit. Along with the many babies born a few weeks prematurely, there were a couple of preemies like Max born on the border of viability. As days turned into weeks, Max endured a roller coaster of progress and setbacks but slowly improved. Nicki and Peter had plenty of scares. Like the time Max had to undergo surgery to repair an artery in his heart. Another week, he got an infection and had to have a spinal tap. But over time, ounce by ounce, he gained weight. After several weeks, he graduated to a nasal breathing tube. "I almost cried the day he came off the ventilator," says nurse Mahoney, who regularly checked on Max's progress, even if she was assigned to another baby. "No one expected him to get that far." At two months, he was sucking on a pacifier and wearing baby clothes decorated with dancing bears. Finally he slept in a crib rather than an incubator.

It took 112 days before Max could be discharged. He weighed 6 pounds. It was still unclear whether or not he would develop learning disabilities or suffer delays in walking or talking. But he was ready to go home.

On their last trip to the NICU, Nicki and Peter brought a homecoming outfit for Max and a car seat, as if they were parents of a newborn, not a four-month-old. Peter videotaped the nurses and doctors, as well as the NICU that had been Max's home for so long. "Peter used to joke that he hoped our children would have my genes," says Nicki, whose family members have all been exceedingly bright. "Of course, I think about this stuff and the problems Max may have. But we've wanted a baby for a long time. We love him to death. We're just so glad to have him and that he's alive."

When Nicki looks back on her journey, she can't imagine doing it differently. Desperate to become a mother, she did what medical technology offered her. And the more times she underwent IVF, the bigger gambles she was willing to take. "I think everyone who does IVF should take a tour of the NICU first," she says. "But we'd had so many failures. Do I regret what we did? No. But will I ever get over losing Seth? No."

Not long ago, Nicki met someone who had a similar story—at least in its beginnings. The woman had endured in vitro and was pregnant with twins. Everyone was thrilled for her. Nicki felt something else. "I had a strange reaction," she says. "I thought, I hope you make it."

2

In Vitro Fertilization Brings Joy to Infertile Couples

Chaya Raizel Breger

Chaya Raizel Breger is a labor coach and lives in Jerusalem with her family.

The author discovers she cannot have children naturally because of cancer surgery years earlier. Despite a reluctance to undergo hormone injections and invasive procedures, she decides to try in vitro fertilization as a last resort. After months of anticipation, she rejoices over the birth of her child.

The news that high-tech fertility treatment was our only option came as a terrible shock to me and my husband. That was the verdict of the very first doctor we consulted, a year after we were married. Such drastic intervention with drugs and surgery seemed more than distasteful; it seemed to go against the very essence of how we lived and approached life. It did not fit in with my image of us as a down-to-earth, ecologically oriented couple. Dismayed, we pushed off additional testing. When I had spurts of willingness to seek other medical opinions, we saw more doctors and underwent more invasive tests, all with the same conclusion: my ovaries were too far away from the fallopian tubes. But surely, I reasoned, G-d who parted the Red Sea could help a microscopic egg transverse an extra few inches?

Each anniversary marked another year without children. Yet

I was wary of tampering with my body and afraid of exposure to powerful, hormonal drugs. I was, for so many years, so careful with what I ate and drank, consciously avoiding many known carcinogens. How could I risk the side effects of Pergonal, Metrodine and Corigon, if anyone even knew what exactly the risks were? How easily I remembered my vulnerability seven years earlier, when I underwent the intensive nine-hour operation that had caused this situation. A team of doctors had entered my room on the 17th floor of Memorial Hospital, overlooking the East River. They had come to give me more details about the exploratory laparotomy that I would endure on the morrow.

> *I was wary of tampering with my body and afraid of exposure to powerful, hormonal drugs.*

". . . Also, we will have a gynecological surgeon participate in the repositioning of your ovaries," added one nurse.

"What?!" I cried in alarm, sitting up straight from my hospital bed. "What are you talking about?"

"It is an important part of the procedure. Didn't anyone tell you?"

"No, nobody told me anything about it!" I sobbed, wanting to escape from this nightmare.

"In case we discover cancer cells in your abdomen, you will need radiation treatment on the lower half of your body. By moving your ovaries away from the lymph glands that would be exposed to radiation, we will be able to protect them from sterilization," she calmly continued.

I did not feel reassured. The whole operation seemed unnecessary to me. Intuitively I sensed that the cancer had not spread beyond the lump in my neck and the tiny, barely perceptible bump under my arm. But in the world of medicine, my intuitive feelings were not established facts that an oncologist could rely on to determine a course of treatment.

The next morning, half an hour before the operation, when I was already in pre-op, the gynecologic surgeon came to meet me. "I heard that you were upset yesterday about the transposition of your ovaries," he began in a kind voice.

I was only 18 at the time. Marriage and family were not uppermost in my immediate life plans. Survival was first. I answered slowly, "I'm all right. I understand. It's OK now."

He spoke softly. "So you are aware that tampering with your ovaries involves a risk? There is a chance that they may not work at all, but it's the chance we have to take, lest the radiation destroy them completely," he added soberly.

Shocked anew, I could not speak. There was nothing to protest. For some mysterious reason this whole experience was meant to be a part of my life.

Looking back, I am grateful that I had radiation and surgery, combining conventional treatment with more holistic, alternative approaches to healing.

I am sure that my wonderful oncologist at Sloan-Kettering [a cancer research hospital in New York] was afraid that I was going to refuse treatment altogether and opt only to pursue experimental, nutritional therapies. The medical staff had reassured me that I would still be able to get pregnant, and I remember how excited my parents and I were the first time I menstruated after that operation.

But now I was married. The years were going by, and I was afraid to start with our only option—in vitro fertilization (IVF). A neighbor was fostering an infant whose fate was being determined in court. I became intrigued with the idea of my husband and I being her parents. When we held her, we discovered how easily we could love her. We thought she was beautiful. One day my friend allowed us to help care for the baby. We changed her diapers, prepared her bottles, fed, held, burped and soothed her. We decided to call the adoption agency immediately to inquire about adopting her. They informed us that there was already a six-year waiting list.

> *We decided to apply our knowledge of holistic methods to the IVF procedure we were about to endure.*

That same week a friend who was also struggling with the challenge of infertility suggested that we both train to be labor coaches. I was horrified with the idea—how depressing it would be, considering our own situation. But Naomi claimed that this was the perfect "in" for us into the whole wonder of pregnancy and birth. "We will have something to say, something to offer," she continued in an effort to convince me. I joined the class.

Meanwhile, back in the States my younger sister, just 19, was soon to become a mother. How brave of her, I thought. What am I waiting for? We have been given only one medical route, yet I am terrified to try it. Maybe it is time to take the plunge. Leave behind my image of myself as a "naturalist." Leave behind perhaps some inner fear of actually becoming a mother. I looked inside myself and wondered what I was afraid of. And I prayed.

> *Ten hours later . . . our beautiful, healthy baby was born at home into our grateful, welcoming arms.*

A month after witnessing the birth of my first client's baby, I told my husband that I felt emotionally ready to visit the IVF Clinic again, not for a consultation but to begin treatment. We decided to apply our knowledge of holistic methods to the IVF procedure we were about to endure. I reread about visualization, a technique that I had used before while coping with the cancer that had directly contributed to our present situation. We hoped that our years of davenning (praying) at the Western Wall (the Kotel), being kvatterim (G-dparents) at brises (ritual circumcision ceremonies) and being prayed for by others would have added up to open the locked gate in shamayim (heaven). We contacted several Rabbis, both for halachic (Jewish Law) guidance and their blessings for success. We asked specific people, especially our parents, to pray for us. We tried to create a supportive network of prayer. Right before we started, I visited the Children's Memorial at Yad Vashem Holocaust Museum in Jerusalem. In the dark, amidst the reflections of a million tiny lights, I pleaded with G-d to send us just one neshama (soul).

When we started the process, I prayerfully visualized each step of the procedure, imagining what was happening in my body: the follicles developing into ripe eggs, the ovaries protected from overstimulation by soothing cool waters, the eggs joyously being fertilized, and a heavenly light guiding and assisting the embryos as they deeply implanted into the welcoming tissue of my womb. There were four embryos at first. Even though a multiple pregnancy would be very difficult and possibly fraught with complications, how could I pray for only one baby and not express concern for the other three potential lives?

The procedure was invasive, with a whole clinic of doctors, nurses, technicians, surgeons, anesthesiologists and assistants participating in our lives. In an attempt to retain some autonomy and privacy, we decided to inject the daily progesterone shots at home. Instead of having to rush in and out of a nurse's office, I did the shots myself and used that time to relax, visualizing myself and my husband in a flower-filled field of the Galilee, beside a crystal clear running river. In my mind's eye, I saw us sitting beneath a pomegranate tree that drooped with the weight of full, ripe fruit. In this Edenic setting, we prayed for healthy children. A soft beam of light surrounded us, and when it receded back to the heavens, we were surrounded by beautiful, cherubic babes.

The days between blood tests were agonizingly slow. I tried to remain calm and optimistic, keeping my mind and body as relaxed as possible. The crucial beta-HCG test came back positive! Our joy was immense. But we still had months to go, with the fear of miscarriage uppermost in our minds. I turned inward, becoming very private as I focused all my energy on maintaining this precious pregnancy for the full nine months. I continued the visualizations, my prayerful imagery, picturing the baby growing within me. When the 40 weeks were complete, on my due date, my waters broke. Ten hours later, with the assistance of a competent midwife, our beautiful, healthy baby was born at home into our grateful, welcoming arms.

3

Commercial Surrogacy Puts Children at Risk

Miranda Devine

Miranda Devine is a columnist with the Sydney Morning Herald *and the* Sun Herald *newspapers in Sydney, Australia.*

Commercial surrogacy allows the rich to purchase babies. In one case, two gay men were able to buy eggs and pay for a surrogate mother for two newborns. While these two men may turn out to be good parents, there is no guarantee that pedophiles will not be able to buy and raise their victims. Since neither the sperm and egg donors nor the surrogate mother in these cases is involved in the child's life, no one with a physical link to the baby is protecting it. This lack of a natural, nurturing link puts the child at greater risk for abuse.

Five days ago [on December 9, 1999], twin babies, a boy named Aspen and a girl named Saffron, were born in California. Thanks to in-vitro fertilisation and relaxed American surrogacy laws, they officially have two fathers and no mother.

The woman who carried them for eight months in her uterus is no biological relation and the woman whose genetic material helped create them was merely engaging in a commercial transaction with 23 of her eggs.

The babies' official fathers, self-made British millionaires Barrie Drewitt, 32, and Tony Barlow, 35, are gay.

They have spent more than $500,000 and four years trying to become parents after being refused permission to adopt a child in Britain. Finally they turned to a Californian surrogacy agency that specialises in providing babies to rich homosexuals.

Now they are listed on Aspen and Saffron's birth certificates as "parent one" and "parent two."

"Aspen is this big strong boy with lots of black hair, and Saffron is so petite and pretty," Barlow told Britain's *Mail on Sunday* newspaper after watching Thursday's birth. "Here were these jewels we couldn't touch, so we both just looked and stared at them."

They are the typical ravings of a proud new dad. The couple have been together for 11 years. But they have come in for much criticism in Britain.

The parents' position

Drewitt told British magazine *Woman's Own* in October [1999]: "We are bound to be criticised because we are gay. But plenty of heterosexual people become parents by mistake and don't even want a child. We're in a long-term stable relationship and we have a strong extended family. Nobody can ever say that these children are not wanted. The kids will be loved as much as any other and perhaps more than a few."

He does have a point. Heterosexuality does not automatically make for good parents. Barlow and Drewitt may be very good parents, far better parents than many women who allow their children to be exposed to a succession of unsuitable men.

It's a fact that the people who pose the most danger to children are the de facto partners of their mothers, men who have no biological link with them and are likely to resent the children because they remind them of the mother's sexual history.

Barlow and Drewitt, on the other hand, have no such hangups. They have dreamed for years of becoming parents. One of them is biologically linked to Aspen and Saffron, since sperm was taken from each man for the procedure (although only one man's sperm was successful). They have the means to get all the help that money can buy.

The dangers of surrogacy

But, still, there is something intrinsically wrong about a process that essentially allows people to buy a baby. The criticism has nothing to do with the sexuality of the parents.

What if the people who go to surrogacy agencies to procure a baby don't have honourable intentions? Who is the moral guardian of these unborn children?

It's difficult enough to protect the children of bad natural parents. But with surrogacy, the instinctive nurturing links between parent and child are deliberately severed.

The egg donor doesn't care about the baby because she never carried the child in her uterus. The woman who gave birth to the baby doesn't care much because it's not her flesh and blood. The sperm donor is equally uninvolved.

> *There is something intrinsically wrong about a process that essentially allows people to buy a baby.*

The ultimate horror of 21st century science is that if you have enough money you can buy a helpless newborn baby and do whatever you like with it in the privacy of your own home. And there is nothing that can stop you.

The Michael Jackson case

If you can believe the latest reports out of the US [United States], that's what the $250 million pop star Michael Jackson has already done. His two children, Prince, 2, and Paris, 19 months, are said to have been conceived with donated sperm and eggs. Jackson's ex-wife Debbie Rowe, was just the "vehicle" to carry them, according to a report in *Star Magazine* [in December 1999].

Rowe, who received a reported $36 million in her divorce settlement, has not touched Paris since she was born, and has only held Prince four times, including once for a cozy family photograph to scotch rumours that the marriage was a sham.

The magazine also said that Jackson, 41, who is said to bleach his skin, didn't use his own sperm because he wanted his children to be white. He also requested donated eggs because he didn't want Rowe to establish a bond with the children. Jackson's agents have denied the story.

But what is undisputed is the fact Jackson has monopolised the children since birth. "He feeds [Prince], he changes his diapers, he reads to him and he sings to him, he takes naps with him," Rowe said in a TV interview [in 1998]. "I don't need to be there because I would have nothing to do."

This is a man whose career was almost destroyed by allegations he sexually assaulted a 13-year-old boy, to whom he later paid a reported $40 million to settle a civil suit over the allegations, all the while protesting his innocence.

"Children love me and I love them," Jackson said at the time. "They want to be with me. Anyone can come into my bed. Nobody wonders why kids sleep over at my house. It is all moral and it is all pure."

Michael Jackson may be all moral and pure but there are plenty of others who aren't.

What if jailed paedophile Philip Bell, at the height of his fortune, had decided that picking up pre-pubescent boys at Palm Beach was too risky? Instead, he would grow his own boys. What a nightmare.

4

Commercial Surrogacy Benefits Childless Couples

Kim Cotton

Kim Cotton carried Britain's first surrogate baby in 1985 and founded COTS (Childlessness Overcome Through Surrogacy), a network that helps match childless couples with potential surrogate mothers. Cotton resigned from the network in 1999.

Medical advances make surrogacy a strong alternative to childlessness. If a couple chooses surrogacy, they should undergo extensive medical and psychological counseling through every phase of the process. Surrogate arrangements with strangers usually work out better than surrogacy within families because in the second situation, the surrogate mother's costs may not be paid or she may feel pressured to accommodate a childless couple. Ideally, all surrogates would be paid for their sacrifice because of the health risks associated with childbirth, and all surrogacy arrangements would be closely monitored by licensed clinics. While the costs may be prohibitive, the benefits of surrogacy are incalculable.

After the birth of Baby Cotton [in 1985]—a surrogate arrangement engineered by a commercial agency operating in the United Kingdom for the first time—a law was rushed through parliament effectively banning commercial surrogacy, but voluntary surrogacy through COTS (Childlessness Overcome Through Surrogacy) flourished.

Kim Cotton, "Surrogacy Should Pay," *British Medical Journal*, vol. 320, April 1, 2000, p. 928. Copyright © 2000 by BMJ Publishing Group, Ltd. Reproduced by permission.

Natural surrogacy was the only option available until the introduction in 1989 of host surrogacy through in vitro fertilisation. This was a tremendous step forward—it established surrogacy as a medical alternative to childlessness. It gave women who previously had no chance, the opportunity to have their own genetic child, albeit through another woman.

With proper screening, both medical and psychological, surrogacy works well. The importance of counselling before, during, and after an arrangement is vital as all parties can avoid the pitfalls if they are made aware of them. Unfortunately, miscarriage occurs all too frequently, so extra support counselling is crucial at this time. It is necessary also when treatment fails, as expectations are unusually high, even though failure rates are clearly acknowledged at the outset.

> *Surrogate mothers should be fully recompensed for their incredible sacrifice.*

It also seems wise to have an independent ethics committee to approve all cases on their individual merits, as sometimes both clinicians and potential parents can lose sight of the most important person in all of this: the baby. If, for instance, the intending mother has a genetic condition which prevents her carrying a pregnancy, is the prognosis good for her to live long enough to raise the child? Pregnancy is only the beginning and a very small part; looking after the child is by far the hardest— it is physically and mentally challenging.

The potential surrogate mother has to have at least one child of her own, so that she has already experienced pregnancy and childbirth for herself. Being less than 37 years of age allows the intending parents the maximum chance of success, as generally fertility tapers off after this age.

Problems and benefits

In my experience, surrogacy within families can be more problematic than with strangers. Expenses rarely change hands, so expectations are not always met, especially on the surrogate mother's side. She often comes away feeling used instead of fulfilled. Counsellors should screen for emotional blackmail. Family members can feel pressurised and obliged to help. Obviously this is not always the case, as some families' lives are greatly enriched by surrogacy.

The quarantine period imposed for HIV also acts as an enforced cooling off period. It allows all parties time to examine whether this is the best solution for them and allows them to get to know one another better—something that has not always happened in the past. . . .

I strongly agree that surrogate mothers should be fully recompensed for their incredible sacrifice. Pregnancy and childbirth are not without personal risk. Many pregnancies are multiple, often requiring a caesarean section. In the ideal world, egg donors and surrogate mothers would be totally altruistic and prolific. But they are not. Who is exploiting whom? Even when treatment fails, clinicians are not accused of exploiting their infertile patients when the cost of in vitro fertilisation and infertility investigations are prohibitive and the money lost in full. A surrogate mother receives payment only on the successful completion of an arrangement. Overall, surrogacy has a 97% success rate, much better odds than in vitro fertilisation.

It's no surprise to learn that most couples do not go on for further treatment after one or two failed cycles, as often they cannot afford to continue. Many will accept second best and opt for the cheaper natural surrogacy, which at present is almost a do it yourself procedure, requiring no medical intervention.

An ideal solution?

It would be ideal to monitor all forms of surrogacy through the provision of treatment by a few, well chosen, licensed in vitro fertilisation units, covering all regions of the country. An all inclusive fee could include counselling and medical screening. Couples requiring surrogacy could pay a fee to register. Potential surrogates would register too, but for no charge, and be carefully matched to the couple. All expenses incurred by the surrogate mother would be paid out of administrative funds held by the clinic, from the couple's registration fee. We could adopt the professionalism of the surrogate agencies in the United States, but not the commercialism.

The only drawback would be the cost. Infertile couples are ordinary people from all walks of life. Many cannot afford to pay their surrogate mother's expenses, let alone the cost of in vitro fertilisation or artificial insemination procedures in a clinic.

Straight surrogacy arrangements go surprisingly well despite the huge hazards attached. I believe infertile couples should have the choice. They can go through a clinic and meet all the protocols imposed and feel safe in the clinicians' hands. Other couples may prefer to take matters into their own hands and feel that they are back in control. They can proceed in their own time, with artificial inseminations taking place in the more intimate surroundings of their own homes or the home of their surrogate mother.

Whichever method they choose, the benefits experienced by all parties after the successful birth and handover of a long awaited surrogate baby are immeasurable.

5

Posthumous Conception Is a Gift

Gaby Vernoff

Gaby Vernoff was the first person to use sperm from a deceased man to conceive a baby.

The author recounts her experiences with posthumous semen retrieval after the accidental death of her husband, Bruce, from an overdose of painkillers. The couple had wanted to have children together, so Gaby, along with Bruce's family, decided to extract and freeze his sperm. On her second attempt at in vitro fertilization, she became pregnant. Gaby gave birth to a healthy girl almost four years after Bruce's death.

I've always felt compassion for women who want a baby so badly that they're willing to go through long, painful, and complicated fertility procedures to conceive. I just never thought I'd be one of them—I'd always assumed that having a baby would be easy for me.

When Bruce and I met, in 1987, we were young and healthy. I had just moved to Los Angeles from Mexico to go to school. I found a job working for Wally and Vidalia Vernoff, Bruce's parents, taking care of their house and helping Vidalia, a high-school Spanish teacher, grade her students' papers. On my first day at work, I met Bruce, and I think I fell in love with him right then. Bruce was such a gentleman, spoke excellent Spanish, and made me feel welcome and at home. Somehow I knew I was going to marry him. Bruce's feelings were slower to surface. It wasn't until about eight months later that our romance blossomed. One night, staring up at the stars, he and I kissed.

Gaby Vernoff, as told to Patt Morrison, "My Husband's Last Gift," *Parents Magazine*, March 2000, p. 143. Copyright © 2000 by Gruner & Jahr USA Publishing. All rights reserved. Reproduced by permission.

I felt weird about living under the same roof as Bruce if we were going to date, so I moved out of the Vernoff home and found another job. We dated for another couple of years and got married on March 20, 1990, in a little chapel in Hollywood.

Bruce and I wanted children, but a month after our wedding, a car accident almost ruined our plans for a family. I broke a rib; Bruce fractured his leg in 11 places. His leg was so badly damaged that his doctors weren't hopeful that they could save it. But Bruce, who worked as a security guard and had always been strong and athletic, couldn't imagine giving up the activities he loved. On family trips to Yosemite National Park, he would climb and hike all day. He was also skilled at martial arts—he even appeared in a low-budget kung fu movie.

> *I didn't want just a baby—I wanted his baby, our baby.*

Bruce started physical therapy, determined to regain full use of his leg. On cold mornings, we'd go to the beach together so he could run on the sand to build up his strength. That was the kind of spirit he had. In his wallet, he always carried a message he got from a fortune cookie. It said, "The greatest pleasure in life is doing things that people say you cannot do."

As Bruce recovered from the five operations needed to repair fractures in his leg, he'd sometimes be in so much pain that he could hardly sleep. He relied heavily on painkillers. Still, he never wanted to give up, lie around, or stop living his normal life.

It took several years, but by 1995, Bruce was off the medication and his leg was much better. He worked as a mail carrier and I went back to studying English. We felt, at last, that this was a good time to start our family.

Keeping our dreams alive

I had an early-morning class on July 3, 1995, and when I got home around noon, I called out to Bruce. He didn't answer. We had slept in separate rooms the night before because Bruce had stayed up late to watch television. I figured he was taking advantage of his day off by sleeping in. I found him lying in bed with the TV still on. When I touched him, though, he was cold and hard. I started crying and screaming, "Bruce! Bruce!" I rubbed his hands frantically to warm them up. I tried to pick him up and move him, but he was so heavy and so cold. Through my tears, I kept yelling, "Get up! Get up!" He didn't answer.

I called my in-laws to say that something was terribly wrong. Then I ran to our next-door neighbors for help, and they called 911.

The coroner later said that Bruce, who was just 35, had accidentally taken a lethal dose of pain medication. He had been off the pills for a long time, but he had strained his muscles a few days before while out climbing. He took the same dose of pills that he had taken shortly after the accident, and his system just couldn't handle it.

After the coroner left, the family sat around crying, stunned. "This can't be happening," we kept saying. I grieved for Bruce and also for the fact that he and I would never have children. "Now all our plans are gone," I said. My sister-in-law, Suzy, tried to comfort me. She told me that she remembered reading somewhere that sperm are viable for a while after death. "I don't know if this would work, but maybe there's a way we could have Bruce's sperm retrieved and keep it as an option," she said. Her suggestion sounded unthinkable at the time, but we were in such shock that I think we grasped at this glimmer of hope, no matter how tiny.

We started calling everybody—family, friends, and neighbors—to find a doctor to help us. Everyone thought the idea was worth a try. Finally, at 1:00 A.M. on the Fourth of July, one day after Bruce died, the phone rang. It was Cappy Rothman, M.D., a urologist who over 20 years before had pioneered the procedure of extracting sperm postmortem and who founded California Cryobank, Inc., a sperm-and-tissue storage facility in Los Angeles. Our family doctor had gotten him out of bed and told him about Bruce's death. "Meet me at the coroner's office at 7:00 A.M.," Dr. Rothman said. The next morning, while we sat there at the county coroner's office, about 30 hours after Bruce died, Dr. Rothman retrieved his sperm—five little vials. He put them in a cooler and took them to the sperm bank to be frozen.

Being a 28-year-old widow was almost too much to bear. I wanted to try to have Bruce's baby right away. We had planned on starting a family now anyway. But my in-laws made me see the importance of a mourning period. I was young, and they were afraid that I might have regrets later. Dr. Rothman, in fact, said that though he'd done more than a dozen such harvests, no family had ever decided to use the sperm later. Everyone wanted me to be really sure about this.

Not just any baby

For the first year after Bruce died, I simply lived day to day. I'd get up in the morning, and the first thing I'd think of was my husband. In the middle of the night, I'd wake up and think of him. I couldn't even go to the movies, because seeing another couple kissing or touching would make tears roll down my cheeks.

I saw a psychologist for a while, and about 18 months after Bruce's death, I felt ready to get pregnant. My doctors decided I was in good emotional shape, and I was eager to make our dream happen. Every day for two weeks before the fertilization, I injected myself with painful shots of hormones. Doctors thawed some of Bruce's sperm, looking for any that might be moving. They harvested my eggs and fertilized them, then implanted three embryos two weeks later. Then we waited. I was sure I was going to get pregnant immediately. I thought, I'm young and in good health; this should be simple. But a month later, we discovered that none of the embryos had taken. The news hurt almost as much as when I'd lost Bruce. Worse still, four of the five vials of sperm had been used.

> **"** *I think Bruce would be so happy about this. It just hurts, though, that he's not here to see our little girl.* **"**

Many people asked me, Why go through all this trouble? Friends and relatives reminded me that I might meet someone else, remarry, and have a baby then. But I did all this because I was in love with Bruce. We had planned a family together. I didn't want just *a* baby—I wanted *his* baby, *our* baby. Believing that I could still have Bruce's child made me happy, and most people I knew understood and supported that. When I decided to save the sperm, I knew a baby wouldn't bring my husband back, but it could bring back part of him.

Of course, we never stored Bruce's sperm when he was alive—we never thought we'd need it. Some medical ethicists, therefore, are quick to point out that I never had Bruce's permission to harvest his sperm and use it. All I can say is that Bruce and I talked a lot about having kids, and he definitely wanted them. We were a couple, a married couple, and we had plans to have a baby. They were *our* plans. That was permission enough.

Life after death

More than a year after the first in vitro attempt, I went for one last chance. With only one vial of sperm left, I tried not to get my hopes up. This time, though, we had the help of another doctor, Paul Turek, M.D., from the University of California at San Francisco, who had developed an innovative technique for identifying living sperm, even if they weren't moving. He found enough viable sperm to fertilize two of my eggs, and miraculously, one of the embryos took. I was glowing with absolute joy my entire pregnancy.

During my labor and delivery last March, Vidalia and Suzy were my coaches. Suzy had a big picture of Bruce, a 16-by-20-inch blowup, made for the delivery room, so in a way, he was there with me the whole time. An epidural helped to ease the pain of more than 12 hours of contractions, and at 10:13 P.M., our daughter was finally born. Cradling my newborn in my arms, I felt I'd been given a precious gift. I named her Brandalynn Danielle so she would have the same initials as her daddy, Bruce David.

I think Bruce would be so happy about this. It just hurts, though, that he's not here to see our little girl. Brandalynn is toddling and babbling now, smiles at everybody, and loves animals—just as Bruce did. She even makes little gestures with her mouth like him. I can only imagine how Bruce would hold her and talk to her. Still, this baby is going to be raised by a family of loving grandparents, uncles, aunts, and cousins.

When Brandalynn is old enough to ask where she came from, I'll tell her that she's special. I'll tell her that she's a little miracle, because her father and I and the entire family wanted to have a baby just like her to love but almost couldn't. Through science and the grace of God, though, she came into our world, defying all odds. I was surprised—and still am—by all the attention we received, but I think it's because this story gives people hope. Brandalynn is living proof of that fortune-cookie message her father lived by—that the greatest joy comes from doing what others say is impossible.

6

Posthumous Conception Without Consent Is Unethical

R.D. Orr and Mark Siegler

R.D. Orr is the director of ethics at Fletcher Allen Health Care at the University of Vermont College of Medicine. Mark Siegler is the director of the MacLean Center for Clinical Medical Ethics, Pritzker School of Medicine at the University of Chicago.

New reproductive technologies make posthumous conception—implanting sperm from a dead man into a woman's womb—a reality that requires discussion and debate. Several ethical guidelines should be followed before allowing posthumous conception to take place. First, the dead man's body must be respected, which means that semen cannot be retrieved unless it is clear that the man would have consented to the procedure without coercion. Next, physicians must consider the welfare of the potential child before assisting in a procedure to help a woman become pregnant using the semen of her deceased partner. For example, they would likely refuse to do artificial insemination on a woman carrying a dominant gene for a serious disease. Ultimately, unless a man expressly wanted his widow to bear his children after his death, posthumous conception is unethical.

There have been sporadic reports of babies born after posthumous conception since the technology became available 50 years ago. Most commonly, a young man has an illness which threatens his fertility or his life—for example, testicular carcinoma. He has some of his semen frozen in order to impregnate his wife in case he should become sterile or to impregnate his widow if he should not survive. In these relatively uncommon cases of posthumous conception, legal questions have been raised about inheritance and eligibility for survivor benefits. Few questions have been raised, however, about the ethics of the procedure because the semen was donated voluntarily, before death, with the expressed intent of use after death.

Retrieval of viable sperm after death . . . raises significantly different issues. It has been reported in the popular press that a baby has been born using posthumous sperm collection after a young man died unexpectedly from an allergic reaction. At his wife's request, sperm was collected 30 hours after death. Fifteen months later his sperm were used to impregnate his widow.

> *In Western society, there is no universal prohibition of posthumous gamete retrieval or posthumous in vitro fertilisation.*

Such requests are infrequent; 82 were reported in the US in a 1997 study, of which about one-third were honoured. Reported successes will likely encourage more requests. In addition, the advent of intracytoplasmic sperm injection (ICSI) now makes it possible to fertilise an egg in the laboratory using a single sperm rather than the several cubic centimetres of semen required for artificial insemination. After describing the technical feasibility of sperm retrieval after death, however, a standard textbook of urology concludes: "the ethical appropriateness of such retrieval is the most important issue surrounding its use".

An identical endpoint—the dramatic birth of a dead man's baby—makes voluntary sperm donation before death and involuntary sperm retrieval after death seem only a small step apart. The difference between these two procedures is not, however, a small step.

In Western society, there is no universal prohibition of posthumous gamete retrieval or posthumous in vitro fertilisation. However, recently reported successes have prompted discussion in the popular press. These practices raise at least three significant ethical questions. First, the method of sperm collection raises issues about respectful treatment of a dead body. Second, there is the issue of consent, important in all invasive procedures. Third is the issue of the welfare of the child to be. We will present two cases which highlight these issues.

A case with no consent

A 28 year old man had been married for six years and he and his wife were childless. He became depressed after a marital separation three months ago. Two weeks ago he started antidepressant medication, but today he was brought to the hospital by paramedics with a self inflicted gunshot wound to his head. Six hours later he was pronounced dead in the intensive care unit. He is the only child of his parents. Just before he died, they asked the intensive care physician to arrange for sperm retrieval after his death so that they might have a grandchild. They said they are certain he would want his biological line continued, and they thought his estranged wife, who had been contemplating reconciliation, would be willing to have his child.

A clinical ethics consultant was asked to review the situation and make recommendations. After talking with the parents and widow, he was unable to elicit any substantiating evidence that the man would want his widow to bear his child. He recommended against the requested sperm retrieval.

A case with implied consent

A 36 year old previously healthy man was admitted with pneumonia. He developed adult respiratory distress syndrome requiring assisted ventilation. After 14 days of aggressive treatment, he became obtunded and developed multiorgan system failure, and his wife was informed that he would not survive. She asked if semen could be collected so that she might yet have his child. An ethics consultation was requested.

They had been trying unsuccessfully to have a child for over 10 years. Two months before this illness they saw an infertility specialist and were to begin in vitro fertilisation with her next menstrual cycle. Although this history indicated his desire to become a father, this alone could not be construed as consent for either sperm collection in this circumstance of impending death or for posthumous collection. The uncertainty of whether he would want his wife to be a single mother after his death was troublesome, and his views on the well-being of a child raised by a single parent were likewise unknown. The wife believed that he would want this, but they had never discussed the possibility. This presumption was supported by his sister who had talked with him about his intense desire to have children in order to continue his family name. But is a wife's intense desire for her husband's offspring morally relevant, and if it is, is it sufficient to justify the removal of semen without his explicit consent? His physicians, nurses and ethics consultant believed the available information adequately supported his wife's expression of his presumed wishes. Within one hour of his death, his epididymides were removed and frozen.

Respect for the deceased person

Metaphysically, the person disappears from his or her body at death, but the dead body continues to command respect. This nearly universal respect for the dead body can be observed as the evening news brings images of grieving survivors searching for the bodies of their loved ones who have been lost at the scene of natural disasters around the world. In most cultures, there seems to be an innate drive to recover bodies so they may be given proper burial. Though individuals in some cultures may believe that organs and physical structures of the once living are no longer important, this is distinctly uncommon in Western society. At the same time, this almost sacred respect for the dead body is not held to be absolute. Most people in Western society accept that there are some exceptions when the body may be disturbed before being buried—for example, for postmortem examinations, and for organ or tissue retrieval for transplantation. Other uses of the dead body have led to considerable controversy—for example, the practising of medical procedures by medical trainees.

Postmortem examination has been practised at least since the time of Julius Caesar in order to learn the cause of death, to further understand the pathology or pathophysiology of disease, or for medicolegal reasons. While many individuals still have a natural revulsion to the idea of cutting, opening, and inspecting the dead body, the potential benefits to the medical profession, the family, or to society as a whole have generally overcome this resistance as long as the autopsy procedure is carried out with the maximum possible respect for the departed person.

For over 30 years, after informed consent by all parties, organs and tissue have been retrieved from recently dead bodies and have been used to save thousands of lives. The concept of death using neurologic criteria, developed primarily to allow the timely retrieval of usable organs, has not, however, been universally accepted, and continues to be the subject of controversy. The drive to overcome the current shortage of organs for transplant has led to the development of new techniques for retrieval of organs from "non-heart-beating cadaver donors", with not-unexpected criticism. But overall, a majority of individuals in Western society believe the good achieved by the donation of organs and tissues outweighs initial concerns about the desecration of the dead body. In spite of this consensus, there has been some aesthetic, cultural, and religious resistance to the practice of organ retrieval and transplantation as an enterprise. In addition, some who accept organ transplantation have specific reservations about the disrespectful treatment of dead bodies in some circumstance. For example, [scholar J.E.] Frader has criticised the practice of providing artificial support for a pregnant corpse in order to bring the gestating fetus to viability, maintaining that this represents a profound disrespect for the dead body.

> *The practice of retrieving sperm from men in coma or recently dead . . . has been criticised as 'perilously close to rape.'*

The responsibility for disposition of the dead body has traditionally been given to the family, or when no family is available, to the church or the state. Consent is almost always sought from the family or the state before doing procedures which would otherwise be deemed disrespectful. While occasionally a medicolegal postmortem examination is authorised by the state over the objection of family, most autopsies are preceded by the consent of the family. Likewise, organs are not removed for transplantation without the consent of the family. It is an interesting commentary on contemporary society that even when a person has specifically documented in writing that he or she wants to be an organ donor, transplant teams are unwilling to retrieve organs without explicit agreement from the family. At least in this situation, the wishes of the family are honoured over the explicit wishes of the deceased, perhaps out of concern for liability. But the reverse is not true. If a patient had specifically declined to be an organ donor, transplant teams are unwilling to retrieve organs after his death even with an impassioned plea from his family.

The issues of utility and consent have also dominated discussion of practising medical techniques on newly dead bodies. While a strong case has been made for the utility of such an approach, it has been called "unlawful and unethical" if it is done without family consent. This example of treating dead bodies in less than a respectful way has often been carried out in secret and has clearly not achieved societal acceptance as have autopsy and organ retrieval.

The majority acceptance of some instances of trespassing the integrity of a dead body in order to benefit others indicates that the strong societal mandate to show respect for a dead body is not inviolable. The practice of retrieving sperm from men in coma or recently dead has not, however, been similarly accepted. This practice has been criticised as "perilously close to rape" by law professor L.B. Andrews.

Determining consent

The ethical concept of valid consent and the legal doctrine of informed consent have become firmly established as foundational in the practice of modern medicine. Ethically valid consent has three components: (1) the patient must have decision making capacity; (2) he must be given adequate information, and (3) then he must give voluntary consent without coercion.

When a patient does not have decisional capacity, consent may be obtained from a proxy. The proxy's "substituted judgment" ought to reflect the decision that the patient would make if able, based on a written advance directive, the patient's previously expressed wishes, or an understanding of his or her values.

In some situations "implied consent" may substitute for a formal consent discussion. Implied consent may sometimes be inferred from the patient's actions. For example, when a man comes to the emergency room (ER) complaining of chest pain and collapses, it can be assumed he wanted treatment. Different still is "presumed consent" which does not depend on a patient's words or actions, but is based on a theory of human goods. It may be presumed that a person unconscious from injuries sustained in a motor vehicle accident would want to be treated. Thus, when substituted judgment is not possible—for example, in a child who has not developed decision making capacity or in an adult who has not made his wishes known, the proxy is allowed to use the lower and more ill defined standard of "best interests".

> *Spousal requests for sperm collection after death should be declined unless there is prior consent or known wishes of the decedent.*

When an emotionally involved third party requests sperm retrieval after death, it might seem desirable to seek the same level of certainty we attempt when making other medical decisions, such as limitation of treatment for patients near the end of life. We could use the same hierarchy of (a) patient's current statement; (b) written advance directive; (c) report of previously stated wishes; (d) recognised values, and (e) presumed best interests. When making limitation of treatment decisions, professionals often experience greater discomfort as we move down this scale of increasing uncertainty, but we cannot avoid making the decisions. We must make the best decision possible in the face of limited information and a particular set of clinical circumstances.

This hierarchy, complex as it is to apply in limitation of treatment decisions, may be even less useful in decisions about sperm collection after death. It is rare for a healthy young man to anticipate life-threatening illness, and even more rare for him to contemplate or discuss whether he would want his sperm to be collected after death so that his widow could bear his child. In addition, such a decision, like many end-of-life decisions, is not just about his life. It has major implications for his wife's future and for the future of his potential progeny.

The legal doctrine of informed consent is based on the ethical principle of autonomy. But this right to self determination should not be misinterpreted to mean that whatever the patient wants should be done. Autonomy is a bounded liberty. Though the patient's negative right to be left alone is nearly absolute, the positive right to have what one wants is clearly not absolute. While a patient may request any treatment desired or imagined, the physician, also an autonomous moral agent, is free to decline a treatment he or she believes is not medically indicated, or is felt to be not in the patient's best interests. A patient's request to forgo or stop dialysis when he finds it disproportionately burdensome should almost always be honoured. On the other hand, a request for narcotics to treat chronic tension headaches should not be honoured if the physician believes an alternative treatment is more appropriate.

The child's welfare

This recognition that the physician has an obligation to do only beneficial procedures and to decline those which are potentially harmful raises the question "who is the patient in posthumous sperm collection"? Does the physician also have a responsibility to decline procedures which may be harmful to a future individual or future generation?

The Human Embryology and Fertilisation Authority of Great Britain requires physicians who provide assisted reproductive technology services to consider the welfare of the potential child before making a decision to proceed. Most physicians would decline to do artificial insemination for a woman who carries a dominant gene for a lethal condition. Some decline to provide services to single women based on studies showing children of single parents do not do as well as children with both parents.

A decision to participate (or not) in helping a woman achieve a pregnancy using the semen of her deceased partner, whether voluntarily frozen for that purpose before death or retrieved posthumously, should consider the welfare of the future child. This calculation is exceedingly difficult, and the conclusion may vary depending on the social circumstances and on personal values. But the issue of the child's welfare cannot be overlooked.

Legal issues

The development of new technology often raises ethical questions about its use. Sometimes these "should we . . . ?" questions seem to be settled by statutory or case law, but usually only after an extended time of legal uncertainty. For example, death defined by neurologic criteria was first proposed in 1968, but settlement of the legal uncertainties did not begin in the US until the proposal for a Uniform Determination of Death Act in 1981. While legislative or judicial determinations often give an imprimatur to a particular action, this does not always fully answer the ethical questions.

There has been some legislative and judicial activity on issues of the status of frozen embryos, parentage after the use of anonymous or designated donated sperm, inheritance after posthumous conception, and other related issues. According to a recent review, however, there have been no laws or cases which give clear guidance about posthumous sperm collection. Based on existing standards of consent, the authors conclude that spousal requests for sperm collection after death should be declined unless there is prior consent or known wishes of the decedent. Their interpretation of the legal climate focuses on the intent of the man, but does not address the issues of treatment of the dead body or the well-being of the potential child.

Applying the ethics of semen retrieval

How should we view a request for sperm collection after death? Does it resemble the family's right to give permission for procedures after death such as autopsy, organ donation, and practising medical technology? If so, can we honour family requests for this procedure? Or might the welfare of the potential child be an overriding consideration?

Although the sperm retrieval procedure itself is far less invasive, destructive, or disfiguring than is an autopsy, the invasiveness seems less important than the man's preferences and the long term consequences for the woman and the child. Autopsy and organ retrieval have more immediate consequence to the dead body, but very little ongoing consequence to the deceased or his family. But sperm retrieval has major consequences for his family and also for his own legacy. In our view, there is a difference in kind between autopsy and organ retrieval on the one hand, and sperm retrieval. Giving consent for autopsy or for organ retrieval for transplantation is giving to benefit others. But requesting sperm retrieval after death without the consent of the dead man is not the same; in fact it is not giving at all—it is instead taking, because its aim is to benefit the person making the request. While retrieval of organs after death without the explicit consent of the decedent is likewise taking, it is different in that the family who is giving consent is altruistically giving the organs for someone else's benefit. The parents or woman who request sperm retrieval after death without the explicit consent of the dead man are making a request for their own benefit. Thus, proxy "consent" in this situation is not consent at all.

In our view, if a man had steadfastly refused to have a child while alive, it would be ethically wrong to honour a request to retrieve his sperm for use after his death. At the other extreme, if we had a clear written or verbal statement from him that he would want to father a child after his death, it might be justifiable to assist this endeavour. If, however, as will likely be the situation in most cases, we do not know his wishes, we must rely on the best available information. In our view, it would usually be appropriate to decline such requests. This stance of non-retrieval without the patient's prior consent or known wishes is supported by the American Society of Reproductive Medicine. They go on to say that "such requests pose judgmental questions that should be answered within the context of the individual circumstances and applicable state laws". While this decision might intensify the grief of the widow, and the poignancy of this refusal would seem to heighten the tragedy of his death, it is the ethically most defensible position based on the presumed rights of the dead or dying patient.

Even with consent, how strongly should we consider a man's stated desire to produce offspring or preserve his family name? While the strength of this desire is clearly evident in many discussions of infertility, it is also true that the desires of many infertile couples can be met through adoption. Thus, the use of requested technology is not always needed to satisfy such desires, and some would say the availability of such alternatives make the use of technology unjustified.

In case 1 above, the lack of consent and lack of knowledge of the man's wishes led appropriately to a refusal to comply with the request. In case 2, there was likewise no consent. His willingness to undergo infertility testing and their plan to pursue in vitro fertilisation suggests that this man had a strong desire to have a child. While this evidence gave some guidance to his medical professionals, it provided no indication of his wishes about his wife having his child after his death. Although she was probably in a position to know his wishes better than anyone else, her own self interest could have clouded her understanding of what his wishes would have been in circumstances that he never discussed and probably never contemplated. His sister's statement lent some support to his wife's contention, but this is still not as definitive as if he had made an explicit statement. The decision to honour her request was thus not clear cut, but was a marginal judgment call.

A request for sperm retrieval after death should not be honoured unless there is convincing evidence that the dead man would want his widow to carry and bear his posthumously conceived offspring. Even when consent is available, professionals should also consider the welfare of the potential child. The evidentiary standards for such a decision are difficult to define and far from clear.

7

Human Cloning Should Be Banned

Michael A. Goldman

Michael A. Goldman is a biology professor at San Francisco State University and has written op-eds for the New York Times *and the* Wall Street Journal.

The pursuit of human cloning is dangerous and should be illegal. First, cloning technology cannot produce an exact duplicate of a human being. Therefore, people who hope that cloning will replace a lost loved one are deceived. Second, cloning is not an ethical solution for couples with infertility problems because if infertility is genetically based, the problem could be passed onto the new generation. In addition, couples could consider adopting one of the many children without loving families rather than resorting to extreme reproductive measures such as cloning. A cloned human faces medical risks such as an increased likelihood of birth defects and disease. It is not fair for parents to risk having cloned children who are more likely to suffer than those conceived under normal circumstances.

The advent of cloning animals from adult cells, and the possible application of this technique to humans, have engendered much debate. In combination with recombinant DNA technology[1] and embryonic stem-cell[2] methodology, cloning is ushering in a staggering new millennium in medicine. I strongly advocate the experimental use of very early embryos (less than two weeks, long before the nervous system is formed) for production of embryonic stem cells and for conducting basic research on the early development of humans. However, there are no scientific grounds for pursuing the use of cloning to produce a human child.

Cloning by somatic nuclear transfer is the introduction of the nucleus of a cell obtained from an existing individual into an egg cell (oocyte) from which the original nucleus has been removed. The egg subsequently begins cell division, under the direction of the introduced nucleus, producing a multicellular embryo that is the genetic twin, or clone, of the nuclear donor. From this very early embryo, scientists can produce embryonic stem cells, isolate cells to learn about genetics and development or attempt to rear an individual to adulthood. Carried to its end point, this is the technology that produced Dolly the sheep [the first cloned animal], an achievement that astounded scientists and the public alike. But the use of this technology to produce a human child is both undesirable and unreasonable at this time.

The reasons for human cloning

First, consider the reasons for producing a cloned human. We may think that a particular individual is exceptionally talented, or exceptionally pretty, and should be perpetuated. We may have lost a loved one and strongly desire to replace this person. Such thinking is fueled by a serious misunderstanding of what it means to be a genetic clone. It is very clear that an individual is a product of its environment as well as its genetic makeup and that a cloned individual may differ quite significantly from the "prototype." In addition, a clone would not share the same cytoplasmic factors, such as mitochondrial DNA, unless the egg donor and the prototype were the same. Thus, the idea that we can duplicate a person by producing a genetic clone is biologically unsound.

1. Recombinant DNA technology is "a body of techniques for cutting apart and splicing together different pieces of DNA," according to the National Institutes of Health.　2. Human embryonic stem cells are cells that come from the inner cell mass of an early embryo (four to five days old). They are capable of turning into any of the more than 200 known types of cells in the human body.

Treatment of infertility is one application that deserves serious consideration as a legitimate reason for wanting to produce a clone. A couple unable to conceive a child may want a
child genetically related to, or identical to, at least one of them.
The psychological imperative to pass on one's genes is a sensi-
tive issue. But that imperative is to produce children who have
half of our own genetic material, not children who are genetically identical to us. If infertility is in part genetically based, we
may be passing on the infertility problem to a new generation.
Fertility treatments abound which also are alternatives to
cloning. There are strong arguments for adopting the many
children who do not have loving families, rather than using extreme measures to produce genetically identical children.

Secondly, we must consider the practicality of producing a
cloned human. While technological advances are likely, our
present capabilities make the process remarkably inefficient. In
cloning Dolly, [professor and scientist in Scotland] Ian Wilmut
and colleagues after many years of related experiments, used
about 400 eggs. Of these, about 277 actually fused with the
donor nucleus. From these couplets, 29 reached a stage appropriate for implantation into 13 foster mothers, and only one—
Dolly—survived long enough for media coverage. Success rates
with some mammals, such as mice, have been considerably
higher, but none have reached a level we would consider impressive for an optional medical procedure. Different animals,
including humans, are likely to respond differently to the procedures and, paraphrasing what they say about mileage in the
auto industry, "your success rate may even differ."

The risks of human cloning

Thirdly, we should take account of the potential dangers a
cloned human might face. As with any medical procedure,
there is risk. While a certain frequency of miscarriage or birth
defects occurs normally, a slightly elevated rate because of the
manipulations involved in cloning would not be surprising.
And we cannot rule out that there might be a drastic increase
in these complications as a result of cloning. Cloning subverts
the normal process of meiosis, a type of cell division used in
the production of egg and sperm. During this process, chromosomes and genes are shuffled so that new, unique combina-
tions of genetic characteristics result. More importantly, major
errors in the DNA are filtered out as damaged cells fail to com-

plete the process. Thus, the eggs and the sperm that fertilize them have passed a strict quality-control test. Somatic cell nuclei, used in cloning, have not only skipped this step, but have been replicating in the body or in culture, accumulating errors with time. We also know that the genetic material is differentially "marked" by the male and female germlines. Some genes only are expressed if inherited from the father, while other genes only are expressed when inherited from the mother, a phenomenon known as genomic imprinting. It is possible that abnormal gene expression might be seen in cloned embryos. The problems outlined here are possible reasons that the efficiency of cloning is relatively low, and this might be a biological barrier that we will never be able to cross.

> *There are no scientific grounds for pursuing the use of cloning to produce a human child.*

The most exciting thing that scientists learned about developmental biology from cloning Dolly might also be one of the most ominous. Somatic cells—those we see in adults—are said to be "differentiated." Somatic cells have specialized to express only a small subset of their 50,000–100,000 genes. Before Dolly was cloned, we thought that this differentiation process was irreversible—once differentiated, a nucleus could not go back and produce a wide variety of other types of cells. Further, adult somatic cells do not divide as efficiently as the cells of early embryos. The cultured breast epithelial cells that were the source of the nucleus that produced Dolly showed us that these two problems do not present an absolute barrier to cloning. But we cannot rule out the possibility that the one in 277 or so fused cells that were successful just happened to be a little atypical. These cells might have been less specialized or more capable of cell division than the rest. Cancerous or precancerous cells may differ from normal cells in their production of certain specialized gene products and in their capacity to undergo continued cell division. Dolly seems quite healthy, but she could have an elevated risk of cancer. The first cloned human might come from an exceptional cell, leaving the newborn on the brink of this grave affliction.

In addition, there could be complications that would appear only later in life. Human cells are limited to about 50 cell divisions, . . . stalked by a relentless internal clock that operates in part as the chipping away of the ends of chromosomes called telomeres. The clock is reset in the process of sexual reproduction. But Dolly skipped this process—she was cloned from a somatic cell rather than from the union of egg and sperm. Scientists have shown that her telomeres are shorter than those of similar-aged ewes, suggesting that she might age prematurely.[3] In contrast, a group of cloned calves had telomeres that were longer than usual, suggesting the possibility of an extended life span. But longer telomeres are also sometimes seen in cancer cells. Do parents want to risk, knowingly, having a child whose life span will be limited because of the fertility treatment they undertook?

> *Rightly or wrongly, we do not use high-risk, unproven medical treatments, even in terminal cases.*

Finally, we should consider the emotional well-being of the cloned child. If a child were to learn that he had been cloned for specific purposes, such as the ability to play the piano, he might face unreasonable expectations. He might question his existence as an individual, his autonomy. Was he a product manufactured to a specific end, with no rights to make his own decisions? If the prototype had died young of a disease, or even an accident, would the clone think his own fate was sealed? Might the prototype's spouse fall in love with a younger clone? While some of these problems also are faced by identical twins, the latter are not the products of medical intervention.

The promise of stem cell research

I want to emphasize that applications of cloning and related technologies can and should be used to understand and alleviate illness, genetic disease, cancer and the ravages of aging.

---

3. Dolly was euthanized in February 2003, at six years of age because she had developed a progressive lung disease—a condition considered common in sheep twice her age.

Stem cells are cells that are capable of perpetuating by cell division, or of giving rise to a variety of specialized cell types. Our ability to work with embryonic stem cells is one of the most dramatic advances of the last decade. Until very recently, use of federal funds in this essential research has been prohibited because it involves the manipulation of cells from human embryos.

In August [2000] the National Institutes of Health issued guidelines that will permit federally funded scientists to work with embryonic stem cells produced in the laboratories of privately funded scientists. (The stem cells are taken from embryos that were being discarded as a by-product of in vitro fertilization.) While these new guidelines dramatically reverse earlier tight restrictions, the scope of federally funded research will have to be broadened before we can realize the full potential of this research in the public sector. The ability to provide matched tissues for transplantation will require the production of a cloned early embryo for each intended recipient. In other words, before a given individual can receive a tissue transplant there must be a cloned early embryo from one of their cells. However, progress in basic research on gene expression may one day allow us to accomplish similar feats with adult stem cells.

Our analysis must remain theoretical, as we do not yet have data on cloned humans, and the information on other cloned organisms still is very limited. It is just this lack of information, this uncertainty, that should make us proceed with caution. Rightly or wrongly, we do not use high-risk, unproven medical treatments, even in terminal cases. Our first concern in medical intervention is to "do no harm." Why should we be so quick to use a medical procedure that might threaten the very offspring we seek to produce? The reasons for undertaking human cloning are tenuous at best, and alternative treatments for infertility, including adoption, are available. Cloning to produce a child is without scientific merit and has raised serious ethical concerns. Unless and until circumstances change dramatically, it should not be a legal medical option, and it is not a rational medical option.

8

Human Cloning Should Not Be Banned

Peter Singer

Peter Singer is a professor at the University Center for Human Values at Princeton and is the author of numerous books, including Animal Liberation *and* Practical Ethics. *He served as president of the International Association of Bioethics from 1992 to 1995.*

The cloning of an adult sheep has raised an unwarranted alarm about human cloning. People who oppose human cloning wrongly believe that it will change the world dramatically. They are concerned that human cloning will allow a "racist selection of the human race." However, their arguments should focus on banning this one possible consequence of cloning rather than on a complete ban of the technology. Despite the fears of critics, human clones, like identical twins, would be treated as individuals. Cloning should not be stopped without evidence that the cloned human's life would be a terrible one.

I f we were to judge by the amount of attention it has received, from the media, from political leaders and from opinion-makers, the ingenious technical breakthrough that enabled Ian Wilmut to clone an adult sheep would have to be the most momentous scientific event since the first atom bomb was dropped on Hiroshima. It was no surprise that *Time* and *Newsweek* ran cover stories on the issue, nor even that *Newsweek*'s cover featured not the most photographed sheep in history, but three identical human babies standing inside glass laboratory beakers.

The *New York Times*, usually one of the world's more sober newspapers, had articles on cloning virtually every day for more than a week. As [evolutionary biologist] Stephen Jay Gould put it, Dolly [the name of the cloned sheep] became the most famous lamb since John the Baptist designated Jesus the Lamb of God.

The response to cloning

The media justified its coverage by quoting authoritative voices telling the reader that cloning is very scary stuff. The French Minister for Farming, Phillippe Vasseur, said, "Tomorrow someone could well invent sheep with eight feet or chickens with six legs." The German Minister for Science and Research, Juergen Ruettgers, said that cloning of human beings "can never be allowed . . . each and every human being is a unique creation that cannot be the subject of manipulation." Robert Coles, a Harvard child psychiatrist and author, likened cloning to Eastern ideas of reincarnation. The most frightening comment of all came from Nobel Peace Prize winner Joseph Rotblat, who compared Wilmut's breakthrough with the creation of the atom bomb.

Really, Dr. Rotblat? Will cloning cause the instant annihilation of tens of thousands of people, and the slow death from a debilitating illness of thousands more, as the atom bombs dropped on Hiroshima and Nagasaki did? Will cloning ever have the power to destroy all life on earth, as nuclear weapons do today? It hardly seems likely.

> *I doubt that our newly discovered ability to make clones from mature individuals will change the world in any dramatic way.*

Many bioethicists and others who have plenty of expertise in the field reacted in a very similar way. Daniel Callahan, one of the founding fathers of American bioethics, called cloning "a profound threat to what might be called the right to our own identity" and said that a parent who cloned him or herself "robs the child of selfhood." Hiroshi Nakajima, director general of the World Health Organization [WHO], said, "WHO considers the use of cloning for the replication of human individuals to be ethically unacceptable as it would violate some of the basic principles which govern medically assisted procreation. These include respect for the dignity of the human being and protection of the security of human genetic material." This statement was subsequently repeated in a resolution of the Fiftieth World Health Assembly. Frederico Mayor, the head of UNESCO [the United Nations Educational, Scientific and Cultural Organization], was even more sweeping in saying that "Human beings must not be cloned under any circumstances." The European Parliament passed a resolution on cloning which said in its preamble that "the cloning of human beings . . . cannot under any circumstances be justified or tolerated by any society, because it is a serious violation of fundamental human rights and is contrary to the principle of equality of human beings as it permits a eugenic and racist selection of the human race, it offends against human dignity and it requires experimentation on humans. . . ." In the first clause of the resolution, the European Parliament added another ground for prohibiting human cloning. It asserted that "each individual has a right to his or her own genetic identity."

Hasty judgments

In my view, these are hasty, follow-the-crowd judgments. Let us focus first on the prospect of cloning from an adult human being, since this is what set the media alight. I doubt that our newly discovered ability to make clones from mature individuals will change the world in any dramatic way. What is it that we fear? Have we been so carried away by science fiction that we believe that megalomaniacal dictators are going to try to make thousands of clones of themselves? Let us assume that these dictators have the scientific resources at their disposal to do this, and can find the thousands of women necessary to bear their clones. It will still take 18 years for the clones to become adults—and then what? During these 18 years the clones will be growing up in environments totally different from those of the dictators from whom they were cloned. They will, for example, know that they are the clones of a dictator. It is impossible to tell what effect these differences will have on their personality, abilities, and views about the world. Megalomaniacal dictators usually find easier—and much nastier— ways to leave their mark on the world.

The European Parliament resolved that human cloning

must be prohibited because each individual has a right to his or her own genetic identity. It would be hard to find a better example of the absurdity of the current fashion of plucking new rights out of thin air. From where does such a right come? On what is it grounded? And where does it leave identical twins? Does the mere existence of their twin violate their right to their own genetic identity? Could one twin use it as a defense to a charge of murdering his or her twin: "Your Honor, I acted in order to defend my right to my own genetic identity?"

What about the claim that cloning is contrary to the equality of human beings because it permits a eugenic and racist selection of the human race? It is true that cloning does permit this, but so do a host of other techniques. Artificial insemination, for example, is already used to select cattle and other domestic animals for particular characteristics. There is nothing in the technique of artificial insemination that would rule out a similar use in humans. Should we therefore prohibit the use of artificial insemination among humans, for fear that it will be used in a racist or eugenicist way? Sterilization already has been used, not only in Nazi Germany, but also in many other countries, in a racist and eugenicist way. Should we prohibit vasectomies and tubal ligations? Much better, I think, to prohibit specific morally objectionable applications of such techniques.

Since at present in most of the developed world untrammeled free enterprise is a more realistic concern than fascism, perhaps we should worry not about state-promoted racist or eugenic uses of cloning, but rather about movie stars, sporting heroes and Nobel Prize–winning scientists seeking to cash in on their fame by selling their DNA to people who would like to be the parents of their clones.

> *If a few people did give birth to clones of Mick Jagger, Madonna, Michael Jordan or Jane Goodall, would that be such a terrible thing?*

Even if cloning were to become a simple enough technique to make this affordable for some, I doubt that it would ever become widespread. And if a few people did give birth to clones of Mick Jagger, Madonna, Michael Jordan or Jane Goodall, would that be such a terrible thing? We might pity the children, who could be under great pressure to live up to the talents of those from whom they were cloned, but to compare their problems with those of the victims of nuclear weapons, as Rotblat did, is grotesque.

Cloning and identity issues

It is not only politicians and bioethicists who have made comments on these issues that were not well-considered. Research scientists have done no better.

Even Wilmut has said: "I am uncomfortable with copying people, because that would involve not treating them as individuals. And so I posed the question that I would like to ask anybody who is contemplating such a use: 'Do you really believe that you would be able to treat that new person as an individual?'"

Does anyone think that people who are identical twins are generally not treated as individuals?

> *Cloning would eliminate the genetic lottery, and ensure that a future child could be a perfectly matched donor for an existing child.*

Perhaps Wilmut would say that twins are not planned, but there is a special problem with the deliberate creation of a new person who is a clone of an existing person. Such remarks are reminiscent of the storm of criticism that greeted the news, in March 1990, that a Los Angeles couple, Abe and Mary Ayala, were having a baby in the hope—the odds were only one in four—that the child would be a bone marrow donor for their 17-year-old daughter, Anissa, who had leukemia and for whom a two-year search had produced no suitable donor. This, medical ethicists thundered, is using a human being as a mere means! It was wrong, even "outrageous."

Despite the criticism, the Ayalas went ahead, and, luckily for Anissa, the child was a match. Anissa's life was saved, and Marissa, the new addition to the family, though perhaps initially desired instrumentally, soon became a much loved child of the family. If what the Ayalas did was wrong, it seems to have been a remarkable kind of wrong, for it has greatly benefited at least three people—Anissa Ayala and her parents—and it has harmed no one. Indeed, if we can benefit a child by bringing her into existence and doing our best to ensure that she has a happy life in a loving family, that is exactly what the Ayalas have done for Marissa, so arguably it is not three, but four, people who have benefited.

Questions about quality of life

This last question—Do we benefit beings by bringing them into existence, if their lives are not clearly awful?—is generally not raised in debates about cloning humans, yet it is clearly relevant to the ethics of cloning a human being. Are we going to condemn cloning if the life of a cloned human being might be somewhat more troubled than the life of a human being produced by the usual process? Or is cloning wrong only if we can show that the life of the cloned human being would be so bad as not to be worth living?

Think for a moment about the fact that, in every major children's hospital in the developed world, extremely premature newborn infants are being kept alive, thanks to the great skill and dedicated labor of highly trained health care professionals. Yet of any given baby with a birth weight of, shall we say, under 750 grams, we know that, if the baby survives at all, there is a risk of somewhere between 25 percent and 50 percent that it will have a moderate or severe disability. We do not see this as a sufficient reason for not trying to keep the baby alive (although where the disabilities are so severe that the life of the child will clearly be awful, we may do so.) I would suggest that the situation ought to be similar with cloning a human being. In the absence of good evidence that the life of the cloned human would be awful, we cannot justify stopping cloning on the grounds that we are acting in the best interests of the cloned human.

There may be genuine medical grounds for cloning a human being, and a situation like that of the Ayalas could be one of them. Cloning would eliminate the genetic lottery, and ensure that a future child could be a perfectly matched donor for an existing child. Of course, if there was a genetic component to the disease, we might well not want to clone from the existing child, but there may be circumstances in which this problem does not arise. In any case, I don't think we are in a position to make any sweeping declarations about the wrongness of cloning a human being until we have carefully considered such possibilities.

9

Sex Selection Should Be Outlawed

Tom Shakespeare

Tom Shakespeare is the director of outreach for the Policy, Ethics, and Life Sciences Research Institute in the United Kingdom and the author of Rights, Risks, and Responsibilities: New Genetics and Disabled People.

New sperm sorting technologies allow prospective parents to select the sex of their offspring. Critics believe that such sex selection is "playing God" and that it reinforces sex discrimination in cultures where males are valued more than females. Furthermore, the sorting technologies do not always work, resulting in the birth of children who are not the sex the parents wanted. Such children may be resented by their parents and grow up feeling unwanted. Accepting the practice of sex selection could lead to allowing the selection of other traits such as athletic ability or eye color—an unethical practice. Therefore, sex selection should be stopped.

So, you want a baby . . . boy or girl? At the Genetics & IVF Institute in Fairfax, Virginia, prospective parents need no longer leave it to chance. For a few thousand dollars, this clinic will take a sample of sperm, colour its chromosomes with a fluorescent dye, and pass it through a laser instrument to separate Y-carrying "male" sperm from X-carrying "female" sperm. After that it's just a matter of taking the batch you want for artificial insemination.

The method is not illegal in the US, and there would be few, if any, legal barriers to clinics in many other countries offering the same service. Small wonder that what is happening in Fairfax has triggered worldwide debate.

Take Britain, which has been at the forefront of reproductive regulation. Its Human Fertilisation and Embryology Authority forbids IVF [in vitro fertilization] clinics from implanting embryos of one particular sex for purely social reasons. But the watchdog's remit is confined to eggs, embryos, frozen or donated sperm and fertility treatment; it has no powers over "sperm sorting". That is likely to change following [the 2002] launch of a programme of consultation, but in which direction? Should regulators ban sperm sorting? Permit it under licence? Or ease resections on implantation and permit both approaches?

The debate over sex selection

Passions run high. Some see sex selection as a recipe for doctors "playing God", and parents commodifying their children. Others argue that unless actual harm can be proven, the state should not restrict individual choice in this most personal of arenas. I believe the pros and cons of sex selection are more finely balanced than these views admit, but that there are nevertheless some real dangers.

Take the worry about sex selection reinforcing gender discrimination. In some parts of the world many parents already choose the sex of babies, through abortion or infanticide. A 1992 study reported in the *British Medical Journal* estimated that there were then up to 100 million "missing" women who were never born or who perished as infants. A worldwide survey of pre-implantation genetic diagnosis found that in 2001, the technique was used for social sex selection in 9 per cent of cases, mostly in the Middle East.

Fans of sex selection say that proper regulation could ensure it didn't create a gender imbalance. A couple wanting a boy could be paired, via a register, with a couple wanting a girl. Or else sex selection could be limited, as it is in the Fairfax clinic, to "balancing" a family's gender make-up. But such rules would not solve all potential problems.

Some bioethicists argue that couples who strongly desire a particular sex of child may have stereotypical gender views and be more likely to rear the child in a sex-stereotyped way. If a much-desired girl turns out to be a wilful tomboy, what would be the reaction of parents who longed for a dutiful, feminine daughter?

What if sex selection fails?

And what happens when sex selection fails? Sperm sorting, unless it is combined with IVF and pre-implantation genetic diagnosis, is far from foolproof. Even with the Fairfax method, 1 in 10 attempts for a girl produce a boy and 1 in 4 attempts for a boy produce a girl. And IVF itself remains costly and unreliable. If a couple spend a lot of time and money trying for a boy but end up with a girl, or vice versa, there is a danger the child might grow up feeling unwanted.

The libertarian may retort that we all know third or fourth-born children the same sex as their siblings who were only conceived to balance the family. And it's true that sex selection might reduce the overall number of such "unwanted" children, as well as the sizes of families. But couples who try to balance their family the conventional way know that they only have a 50 per cent chance of success, and must surely be open to a child of either sex. Couples with heightened expectations of success might react very differently.

On balance, then, I believe that sperm sorting will in the long run do more harm than good. And this seems doubly true of sex selection via pre-implantation genetic diagnosis. Even if there is no "gene for" intelligence, sporting prowess or artistic talent, few scientists doubt that gene-chip technologies will one day provide considerable information about genetic variations. Letting parents choose embryos on the basis of sex now, for no good medical reason, will make it far harder in future to say no when they ask to choose embryos on the basis of other traits.

A line has to be drawn somewhere, and social sex selection is the right place. Children should be accepted for themselves, not to the extent that they fulfil our wishes and desires. We should be more tolerant of disability and all imperfection, let alone imbalances of sex within a family. As previously with stem cells, [2003's] decision by Britain will have global repercussions. Through an agreement called the Oviedo Convention, European nations have already expressed a consensus against sex selection. Britain's regulators should hold the line.

10

Sex Selection
Should Be Legal

B.M. Dickens

*B.M. Dickens is a professor of health law and policy at the
University of Toronto, Canada.*

The development of reproductive technology that allows
parents to select the sex of their future children has raised
fears that it will promote sexist preferences for boys. Recent legislation in countries including Canada and the
European Union prohibits or restricts sex selection because of such fears. However, studies indicate that most
parents in Western countries have no preference for one
sex or the other. Researchers found that parents were
only interested in sex selection in terms of balancing
their families—having at least one child of each sex. New
reproductive technologies such as preimplantation genetic diagnosis and sperm sorting help a couple select a
child's sex before it is implanted in the womb. These procedures help a woman avoid having repeated pregnancies to try to have children of each sex or even using
abortion as a tool for sex selection. In short, prohibitions
against sex selection are oppressive and wrong.

The urge to select children's sex is not new. The Babylonian
Talmud, a Jewish text completed towards the end of the
fifth century of the Christian era, advises couples on means to
favour the birth of either a male or a female child. The development of amniocentesis alerted the public in the mid-1970s to
the scientific potential for prenatal determination of fetal sex,
and progressive decriminalisation of abortion afforded choice
about continuation of pregnancy. The more recent emergence

B.M. Dickens, "Can Sex Selection Be Ethically Tolerated?" *Journal of Medical
Ethics*, vol. 28, December 2002, p. 335. Copyright © 2002 by BMJ Publishing
Group, Ltd. Reproduced by permission.

of preimplantation genetic diagnosis (PGD)[1] obviates resort to abortion, and improved techniques of sperm sorting[2] and diagnosis permit creation of zygotes that will ensure the sex of a future child.

Growth of biomedical means to select the sex of future children has been accompanied by fear that such means will be employed to favour births of sons, and so perpetuate devaluation of girl children and women's inferior family and social status. A reaction to this fear has been the demand for legal and medical professional prohibition of sex selection techniques. For instance, the Council of Europe's Convention on Human Rights and Biomedicine provides in article 14 that:

> The use of techniques of medically assisted procreation shall not be allowed for the purpose of choosing a future child's sex, except where serious hereditary sex-related disease is to be avoided.

Legislation has been enacted in a number of countries, and proposed in others, to prohibit sex selection on non-medical grounds, such as the Prenatal Diagnostic Techniques (Regulation and Prevention of Misuse) Act, 1994 in India. In Canada, for instance, government draft legislation introduced in May 2002 proposes to make it a crime for any person, for the purpose of creating a human being, knowingly to:

> perform any procedure or provide, prescribe or administer any thing that would ensure or increase the probability that an embryo will be of a particular sex, or that would identify the sex of an in vitro embryo, except to prevent, diagnose or treat a sex linked disorder or disease.

In light of evidence from India, China, and other countries and cultures in which son preference is apparent, many analysts and commentators have envisioned the use of techniques of sex selection only as reinforcing male dominated sexism and women's subordination.

New reproductive techniques and technologies have always triggered fears of unnatural, harmful outcomes, social disruption, and destruction of conventional families. In the mid-

---

1. Preimplantation genetic diagnosis (PGD) "allows genetic analysis to be performed on early embryos prior to implantation and pregnancy," according to the Genetics and IVF Institute.   2. Sperm sorting is the separation of male sperm from female sperm.

1960s, addressing human reproduction by artificial insemination, the gynaecologists Kleegman and Kaufman perceptively observed that:

> Any change in custom or practice in this emotionally charged area has always elicited a response from established custom and law of horrified negation at first; then negation without horror; then slow and gradual curiosity, study, evaluation, and finally a very slow but steady acceptance.

The established custom that was initially, and in some cases is still, horrified at recognition of the potential for effective sex selection of future children was not only that of conservative religion, but also that of some components of organised feminism. By the 1980s, feminism was becoming a politically influential force in Western Europe, North America, Australia, and several other westernised democratic countries. The dilemma posed by sex selected abortion is that many feminists, not all of whom are women, consider choice in abortion to underpin women's moral agency and the defence of their self determination. A leading modern analyst has observed that:

> Whatever the specific reasons are for abortion, most feminists believe that the women concerned are in the best position to judge whether abortion is the appropriate response to pregnancy. Because usually only the woman choosing abortion is properly situated to weigh all the relevant factors, most feminists resist attempts to offer general, abstract rules for determining when abortion is morally justified. . . . Despite the diversity of opinion found among feminists on most other matters, most feminists agree that women must gain full control over their own reproductive lives if they are to free themselves from male dominance.

Sex selected abortion, however, is seen as an instrument and consequence of male dominance that feminists are committed to oppose. It has been observed that "many feminists view any efforts to plan the sex of future children as epitomising sexism". Writing about abortion in 1986, a prominent pro-choice advocate stated: "we believe abortion-for-gender choice is an unqualified moral wrong". Opposition to means of sex selection that are made possible by PGD and sperm sorting avoids the dilemma posed by sex selected abortion, and affords opponents the support of conservative antiabortion agencies, as well as of others committed to the elimination of the pro-male sexism that sex selection is seen to represent.

> *Selection based on sex is clearly sexual, but not necessarily sexist.*

The stereotypical concept that pro-male sexism is inherent in sex selection, rooted in perceptions of pervasive devaluation of girl children, may be contradicted in particular countries, however, by empirical studies. For instance, summarising the conclusion of a comprehensive sociological survey and public presentations, members of the Royal Commission on New Reproductive Technologies in Canada reported in 1993 that:

> The survey revealed that, contrary to what has been found in some other countries, a large majority of Canadians do not prefer children of one sex or the other. Many intervenors . . . assumed that Canadians have a pro-male bias with regard to family composition; we found that this assumption appears to be unfounded.

Interest in sex determination was found to be very low, and concerned only with family balancing. The commissioners reported regarding sex preferences that:

> Preferences were generally seen as unimportant, almost trivial. The survey showed that virtually all prospective parents want, and feel strongly about having, at least one child of each sex.

Nevertheless, invoking perceived feminist values, the commissioners recommended criminalisation of the use of sex selection techniques, which is now proposed in the legislation introduced in May 2002.

This legislation is comparable to that enacted in India in 1994, but raises the ethical issue of whether the social circumstances the legislation is intended to affect are comparable. The ethical principle of justice, considered at a formal or abstract level, requires that like cases be treated alike, and that different cases be treated with due recognition of the difference; that is, it is as unjust and unethical to treat different cases alike as to treat alike cases differently. Male dominance may be comparable in Canada and India, but the evidence is that sex preference between children is different.

There may be the same preference in some families for a firstborn child to be male, but this preference, if offensive to equal priority and opportunity between the sexes, can be addressed by permitting sex selection only for second or subsequent children, rather than by absolute prohibition. Under a limit of this nature, allowing sex selection for purposes of family balancing in countries in which no demonstrable pro-male sex bias exists among prospective parents appears at least ethically neutral and tolerable. Support lies in such tolerance contributing to respect for prospective parents' autonomy. It avoids the harm of compelling a woman's repeated pregnancies until her goal of a family balanced by children of both sexes is achieved, and of abortion of an unplanned pregnancy that may be of a fetus of the balancing sex.

> *Prohibitions are unnecessary and oppressive where there is no sex bias but only a wish to balance a family with children of both sexes.*

Selection based on sex is clearly sexual, but not necessarily sexist. The analogy is with the contrast between racist and racial choice. It is as objectionable for a decision to be sexist as for it to be racist. A racially based decision may be founded, however, on ethical preference, not unethical attribution of inferior status to non-preferred races. For instance, a person's choice to marry a partner of his or her own race may be based on the comfort of common culture and the wish for racially compatible children, not hostility to miscegenation or the belief that races other than one's own are inferior. Similarly, the intention of a couple with a child of one sex to have another child of the other sex is a sexual but not a sexist preference. To suppose that any such choice is necessarily sexist is unjust, and to base laws introducing criminal penalties on such a supposition where the evidence is that an assumption of "a pro-male bias . . . appears to be unfounded" [in the words of the Canadian Royal Commission on New Reproductive Technologies] is both unjust and oppressive.

Where social practice, including that to do with sex selection, is apparently sexist, such as in the environment to which the Indian legislation of 1994 is a response, the ethics of legal prohibition also warrant attention. Since "feminist ethics demands that the effects of any decision on women's lives be a feature of moral discussion and decision making," and focuses "on the need to develop a moral analysis that fits the actual world in which we live", legal prohibition may be examined in that light.

Until their society remedies its son preference, the prohibition of sex selection would seem predominantly to burden women's lives. If wives cannot resist their husbands', and family and religious demands that they deliver sons, they may have to bear successive pregnancies until they do. Early marriage and a quick succession of pregnancies contribute significantly to the risk of maternal mortality and morbidity. A leading gynaecologist has observed that "every woman who gets pregnant is exposed to risk. . . . The risk increases in low resource settings. . . . Risks of pregnancy and childbirth recur with every pregnancy. The lifetime risk of pregnancy and childbirth depends on how many times the woman gets pregnant". Without considering aggravated risks of adolescent pregnancy, a World Health Organisation (WHO) report notes "the disturbing statistics of maternal mortality for developing countries, where women are more than 400 times as likely to die from complications during pregnancy than women in Southern Europe". The risk to unplanned girl children is of early death due to infanticide, malnutrition, or neglect.

Son preference has produced, but might also mitigate, the sex-ratio imbalance. The latest Indian census puts the national sex ratio as 933 females to 1000 males, but only 927 females in the age group under six years old. In Haryana state [in India], moreover, there are 861 girls to 1000 boys, and only 820 females in the under six age group. While ominous for the present generation of children, these figures offer a promise of future redress. If sons wish, as adults, to have their own sons, they need wives. The dearth of prospective wives will, in perhaps short time, enhance the social value of daughters, reversing their vulnerability and the force of male dominance.

Whether or not this promise is realised, attempts to end

son preference by prohibition of sex selection are failing in India, and appear too peripheral on their own, to relieve sex bias, since "the tail cannot wag the dog". Sex bias must be tackled at more fundamental and comprehensive social, economic, political, and legal levels. Prohibitions are unnecessary and oppressive where there is no sex bias but only a wish to balance a family with children of both sexes, and pose risks to women's and girl children's lives and health where bias remains.

11

Reproductive Technology Does Not Need Greater Regulation

Gregory Stock

Gregory Stock is director of the Program on Medicine, Technology, and Society at the School of Medicine at UCLA. He is also the author of Redesigning Humans: Choosing Our Children's Genes.

Overregulating reproductive technologies will jeopardize their potential benefit to humanity. For example, fears over human cloning are unfounded, yet religious and political leaders are pushing for a ban on cloning research that would impede research on diseases such as Parkinson's or diabetes. Many proposals to restrict reproductive technologies are based on false beliefs about their social dangers and should be met with skepticism. Laws against research would force scientists to work in secrecy. The best approach is to avoid imposing rigid laws but cautiously monitor the research, allowing society to benefit from the useful developments science will bring.

We have employed technology extensively to reshape the world around us. For the most part, we are comfortable with this infusion of technology into our lives. But as our power grows, we are turning it back on ourselves to adjust and modify our biology, and this is more worrisome.

As we come to understand our underlying workings more deeply and begin to move beyond mere therapy, many people, fearing we are entering a dangerous realm, think we should try to halt progress until we can figure out the best course. But giving in to our anxieties would be a mistake.

We face two types of risks with emerging medical technologies. The first is obvious: we might injure ourselves. But the second—that too much caution could delay beneficial advances—may endanger far more people. If trends hold, more than 100,000 will die of cancer in Britain in 2015, so there will be direct consequences for many people if some treatments arrive in 2020 instead of 2010.

An overreaction to new technologies

The US Senate's proposed ban on all cloning procedures shows how overblown fears can drive legislation in unfortunate ways. Given that thousands of nuclear-transfer procedures on rhesus monkeys have still not created one viable primate embryo, no responsible scientist would suggest that cloning humans is safe at this time. But does this mean that we need a ban on the procedure when there are already robust institutional mechanisms to discourage reckless human experimentation?

When the procedure becomes feasible and someone somewhere clones a child, will this threaten our way of life? It would be a decade or two more before the procedure became cheap and safe enough to be a clinical option for many couples, and even then its appeal will remain narrow. We will have ample time then to enact any restrictions we wish, so why all the hand-wringing now?

If concern about the safety of children were our major motivation, added attention to childhood nutrition or alcohol abuse in pregnancy would be far more effective uses of our energy. Our fears are not about safety, but rather about values, philosophy and religion, about nightmarish images of the human future. Visions of organ farms and armies of clones evoke memories of reactions a generation ago to the first "test-tube babies" and tell us more about ourselves than about the true challenges ahead.

The danger in overregulation

There is, of course, little immediate danger in banning a nonexistent technology such as human cloning. The real threat is that such bans will begin to inject religion and politics into broad areas of basic biomedical research, thereby delaying the medical advances we all applaud.

As research unravels the processes of life, it will grow ever easier to use this knowledge in challenging ways. But we would have to halt scientific progress itself to stop this. Britain was wise not to outlaw therapeutic cloning of pre-embryos because the action would hardly stop fringe figures such as Severino Antinori,[1] but it would stifle embryonic stem-cell research on Parkinson's, diabetes and other diseases and thereby harm real people with real suffering.

Some argue that safe, reliable procedures that injure no one directly must be carefully regulated to ensure that they have no undesirable social consequences. I disagree. We should be leery about restricting technologies that merely challenge concepts of family or conjure loose notions of social danger because such arguments are easily abused. Sex selection by parents is a good example. Who is injured when a couple chooses to have a girl (or a boy)? The problem of sex imbalances in developing countries is not relevant because no gender imbalances arise from these choices in the West.

> *The US Senate's proposed ban on all cloning procedures shows how overblown fears can drive legislation in unfortunate ways.*

Embargos on victimless procedures are more than an unwarranted intrusion by the state into private life. They drive the practices underground and deny us information about any subtle medical dangers associated with them. We must keep in mind that reproductive technologies are not like nuclear weapons, where one false move can vaporise millions of innocent bystanders. Early users, not bystanders, bear the risks and buy us all valuable information.

The best approach

New technologies emerging from the biotech revolution will be central to our future, revolutionising healthcare, altering the

1. Severino Antinori, an Italian embryologist, announced in November 2002 that he had successfully cloned several humans whose births were due in 2003, but he never produced evidence of the cloned children.

way we have children, changing how we manage our emotions and moods, and perhaps even extending the human lifespan. Some say such claims are extravagant because the technologies will always be too dangerous and ineffectual. If they are right, the present debate will simply fade away.

But the real fear of critics is not that these technologies will fail, but that they will succeed. In this case, tight restrictions will be destructive, for they will not only delay the benefits, they will reserve them for the rich, who find ways to circumvent restrictions.

Our best approach is modest, pragmatic monitoring that responds not to anxieties about the future but to concrete problems. We must avoid rigid, dogmatic legislative forays that will be difficult to alter in response to new data and knowledge. We must legislate cautiously and thoughtfully, balancing the risks of accidents with the risks of lost or delayed benefits.

And we must not forget that our next frontier is not space, but ourselves, and this exploration will not be risk-free. Ultimately, the question will not be how we handle cloning, genetically modified foods or any other specific technology, but whether we continue to embrace the possibilities of the future or pull back in fear, allowing other braver souls elsewhere to take them on.

Organizations to Contact

The editors have compiled the following list of organizations concerned with the issues debated in this book. The descriptions are derived from materials provided by the organizations. All have publications or information available for interested readers. The list was compiled on the date of publication of the present volume; names, addresses, phone and fax numbers, and e-mail addresses may change. Be aware that many organizations take several weeks or longer to respond to inquiries, so allow as much time as possible.

American Society for Reproductive Medicine (ASRM)
1209 Montgomery Hwy., Birmingham, AL 35216
(205) 978-5000 • fax: (205) 978-5005
e-mail: asrm@asrm.org • Web site: www.asrm.org

ASRM is a professional, nonprofit organization providing knowledge and expertise in reproductive medicine and biology. Its Web site offers information for patients on infertility, menopause, contraception, reproductive surgery, endometriosis, and other reproductive disorders, as well as recent news in the field of reproductive medicine. ASRM issues a number of publications, including reports from its ethics committee meetings, its journal *Fertility and Sterility*, and a series of ten-page booklets about reproductive medicine.

Center for Genetics and Society
436 Fourteenth St., Suite 1302, Oakland, CA 94612
(510) 625-0819 • fax: (510) 625-0874
e-mail: info@genetics-and-society.org
Web site: www.genetics-and-society.org

The Center for Genetics and Society is a nonprofit information and public affairs organization that works with scientists and health professionals to encourage responsible uses and effective societal governance of the new human genetic and reproductive technologies. Its Web site provides news, background information, and analysis on issues such as human cloning and eugenics. The center publishes the *Genetic Crossroads* newsletter.

Center for Reproductive Rights
120 Wall St., New York, NY 10005
(917) 637-3600 • fax: (917) 637-3666
e-mail: info@reprorights.org • Web site: www.reprorights.org

The Center for Reproductive Rights is a nonprofit legal advocacy group that promotes and defends women's reproductive rights worldwide. Their Web site provides information about historical women's rights decisions, ongoing projects, and news related to reproductive rights. It publishes a variety of books and reports including its Women of the World series, which details local laws, policies, and quality of life statistics as they relate to women's reproductive health and rights around the world.

Centers for Disease Control and Prevention (CDC)
Reproductive Health Information Source
4770 Buford Hwy. NE, Mail Stop K-20, Atlanta, GA 30341
(770) 488-5200 • fax: (770) 488-6450
e-mail: cdcinfo@cdc.gov • Web site: www.cdc.gov/reproductivehealth

As a division of the U.S. Department of Health and Human Services, this CDC Web site provides statistics and information about reproductive issues and technologies. The CDC publishes many reports, including the *2001 Assisted Reproductive Technology Success Rates: National Summary and Fertility Clinic Reports.*

Council for Responsible Genetics (CRG)
5 Upland Rd., Suite 3, Cambridge, MA 02140
(617) 868-0870 • fax: (617) 491-5344
e-mail: org@gene-watch.org • Web site: www.gene-watch.org

CRG is a nonprofit, nongovernmental organization that seeks to foster public debate about the social, ethical, and environmental implications of genetic technologies. CRG works through the media and concerned citizens to distribute accurate information and represent the public interest on emerging issues in biotechnology. CRG also publishes a bimonthly magazine, *GeneWatch.*

Department of Reproductive Health and Research (RHR)
World Health Organization
1211 Geneva 27, Switzerland
+41 22 791 3372 • fax: +41 22 791 4189
e-mail: reproductivehealth@who.int
Web site: www.who.int/reproductive-health/index.htm

RHR provides information on a variety of topics relating to reproduction worldwide, including sexual and reproductive rights, adolescent sexual and reproductive health, and infertility. RHR publishes two newsletters: *Progress in Reproductive Health Research* and *Safe Motherhood.*

Global Reproductive Health Forum (GRHF)
Harvard School of Public Health
Department of Population and International Health
665 Huntington Ave., Boston, MA 02115
(617) 432-4619
e-mail: jzucker@hsph.harvard.edu
Web site: www.hsph.harvard.edu/grhf

The Global Reproductive Health Forum (GRHF) at Harvard University is an Internet networking project that aims to encourage the proliferation of critical discussions about reproductive health and gender on the net. GRHF provides interactive electronic forums, global discussions, distributes reproductive health and rights materials from a variety of perspectives, as well as maintains an extensive research library.

President's Council on Bioethics
1801 Pennsylvania Ave. NW, Suite 700, Washington, DC 20006
(202) 296-4669
e-mail: info@bioethics.gov • Web site: www.bioethics.gov

The President's Council on Bioethics advises the president on bioethical issues that may emerge as a consequence of advances in biomedical science and technology. This site presents the council's reports in areas of reproductive technology including stem cell research, sex selection, and cloning. The council produces numerous reports and books, including *Monitoring Stem Cell Research* and *Human Cloning and Human Dignity: An Ethical Inquiry.*

Reproductive Health Gateway
e-mail: mdadamo@jhuccp.org • Web site: www.rhgateway.org

Reproductive Health Gateway provides access to relevant, accurate information about reproductive health on the World Wide Web by searching selected Web sites. Their Web site also provides updated news and events about reproduction occurring around the world along with online databases, directories, and a photo library. Dozens of journals and newsletters are available online free of charge, including *JAMA: Journal of the American Medical Association* and *Reproductive Freedom News.*

Resolve, the National Infertility Association
1310 Broadway, Somerville, MA 02144
(888) 623-0744 • fax: (202) 659-1902
e-mail: info@resolve.org • Web site: www.resolve.org

Resolve provides education, advocacy, and support for infertile couples on such issues as egg donation, adoption, and pregnancy. It publishes booklets on infertility as well as *Family Building* magazine.

Bibliography

Books

Lori B. Andrews	*The Clone Age: Adventures in the New World of Reproductive Technology*. New York: Henry Holt, 1999.
Robin Baker	*Sex in the Future: The Reproductive Revolution and How It Will Change Us*. New York: Arcade, 2000.
Gay Becker	*The Elusive Embryo: How Women and Men Approach New Reproductive Technologies*. Berkeley: University of California Press, 2000.
Dena S. Davis	*Genetic Dilemmas: Reproductive Technology, Parental Choices, and Children's Futures*. New York: Routledge, 2001.
Donna L. Dickenson	*Ethical Issues in Maternal-Fetal Medicine*. New York: Cambridge University Press, 2002.
Elizabeth Ettore	*Reproductive Genetics, Gender, and the Body*. New York: Routledge, 2002.
Madelyn Freundlich	*Adoption and Assisted Reproduction*. Washington, DC: Child Welfare League of America, Evan B. Donaldson Adoption Institute, 2001.
Roger Gosden	*Designing Babies: The Brave New World of Reproductive Technology*. New York: W.H. Freeman, 1999.
Gordon Graham	*Genes: A Philosophical Inquiry*. New York: Routledge, 2002.
Arlene Judith Klotzko, ed.	*The Cloning Sourcebook*. New York: Oxford University Press, 2001.
Rachel Kranz	*Reproductive Rights and Technology*. New York: Facts On File, 2002.
Paul Lauritzen, ed.	*Cloning and the Future of Human Embryo Research*. New York: Oxford University Press, 2001.
Caroline Lorbach	*Experiences of Donor Conception: Parents, Offspring, and Donors Through the Years*. Philadelphia: Jessica Kingsley, 2003.
Glenn McGee, ed.	*The Human Cloning Debate*. Berkeley, CA: Berkeley Hills, 2000.
Michael Ruse and Aryne Sheppard, eds.	*Cloning: Responsible Science or Technomadness?* Amherst, NY: Prometheus, 2001.

Maura A. Ryan	*Ethics and Economics of Assisted Reproduction: The Cost of Longing.* Washington, DC: Georgetown University Press, 2001.
Leslie R. Schover and Anthony J. Thomas Jr.	*Overcoming Male Infertility.* New York: J. Wiley, 2000.
Mary Lyndon Shanley	*Making Babies, Making Families: What Matters Most in an Age of Reproductive Technologies, Surrogacy, Adoption, and Same-Sex and Unwed Parents.* Boston: Beacon, 2001.
Dani Singer and Myra Hunter, eds.	*Assisted Human Reproduction: Psychological and Ethical Dilemmas.* London: Whurr, 2003.
Gregory Stock	*Redesigning Humans: Our Inevitable Genetic Future.* Boston: Houghton Mifflin, 2002.
Rosemarie Tong, ed.	*Globalizing Feminist Bioethics: Crosscultural Perspectives.* Boulder, CO: Westview, 2001.
Mary Warnock	*Making Babies: Is There a Right to Have Children?* New York: Oxford University Press, 2002.

Periodicals

Anil Ananthaswamy	"Brave New Babies," *New Scientist,* May 26, 2001.
Andrew Bolt	"Shop of Horrors," *Herald Sun* (Melbourne), August 13, 2001.
C. Cameron and R. Williamson	"Is There an Ethical Difference Between Preimplantation Genetic Diagnosis and Abortion?" *Journal of Medical Ethics,* April 2003.
Deborah Cassrels	"The Baby Makers," *Courier-Mail* (Brisbane), May 15, 1999.
Steve Connor	"Science: Grow Your Own Spare Parts," *Independent* (London), November 10, 2000.
Laura Dempsey	"Infertility: Dashed Hopes . . . Empty Arms," *Dayton Daily News,* December 15, 2002.
Kevin Doran	"Cloning Seems Destined to Destroy More Life than It Produces," *Irish Times* (Dublin), January 2, 2003.
Tom Frame	"The Perils of Surrogate Motherhood," *Quadrant,* June 2003.
Susan Golombok, et al.	"The 'Test-Tube' Generation: Parent-Child Relationships and the Psychological Well-Being of In Vitro Fertilization Children at Adolescence," *Child Development,* March 2001.
Roger Gosden	"New Options for Mothers," *Futurist,* March 2000.
Ronald M. Green	"Should We Be Working Toward Human Cloning for Infertility Treatment?" *Contemporary OB/GYN,* May 2000.

Jerome Groopman — "Holding Cell: Why the Cloning Decision Was Wrong," *New Republic*, August 5, 2002.

Fred Guterl — "To Build a Baby," *Newsweek International*, June 30, 2003.

Anita Hamilton — "Eggs on Ice: A Woman's Fertility Often Peaks Before She's Ready to Have Babies. Does Banking Her Eggs Make Sense?" *Time*, July 1, 2002.

Julie Irwin — "Frozen Embryos Spawn Ethical Debates,"*Cincinnati Enquirer*, August 8, 1999.

Thomas Kennedy — "A Deceptive Good," *Christianity Today*, September 4, 2000.

Marnie Ko — "Worse Odds in a Petri Dish: A New Study Finds Test-Tube Babies Are More Likely to Be Deformed," *Report Newsmagazine*, April 15, 2002.

Nicholas D. Kristof — "The Danger of the New Eugenics," *Gazette* (Montreal), July 5, 2003.

Rebekkah Melchor Logan — "Cloning Debate Takes Cues from Faith," *Asheville (North Carolina) Citizen-Times*, January 18, 2003.

Anne Drapkin Lyerly and Ruth R. Faden — "HIV and Assisted Reproductive Technology: Women and Healthcare Policy," *American Journal of Bioethics*, Winter 2003.

Jeremy Manier — "The Gift of a Lifetime: Infertile Couples Aided by Donated Embryos," *Seattle Times*, September 25, 2002.

Gina Maranto — "Test-Tube Babies and Designer Genes," *Los Angeles Times*, July 25, 2003.

David McCarthy — "Why Sex Selection Should Be Legal," *Journal of Medical Ethics*, October 2001.

R. Timothy Mulcahy — "What Has Dolly Wrought? Allow Research Cloning, Ban Reproductive Cloning," *Wisconsin State Journal*, January 5, 2003.

Shannon Mullen — "In Vitro Fertilization Technology Much Improved After First Birth 25 Years Ago," *Knight Ridder/ Tribune Business News*, July 25, 2003.

Deborah Orr — "The Moral Consequences of This Baby Hunger," *Independent* (London), May 15, 2002.

Erik Parens and Lori P. Knowles — "Reprogenetics and Public Policy: Reflections and Recommendations," *Hastings Center Report*, July/August 2003.

Richard J. Paulson — "Should We Help Women over Fifty Conceive with Donor Eggs?" *Contemporary OB/GYN*, January 2000.

O. Ricardo Pimentel — "Who Says Cloning Isn't God's Plan?" *Arizona Republic*, January 7, 2003.

Laura Purdy
"Empowerment or Danger," *Forum for Applied Research and Public Policy*, Spring 2000.

Elizabeth Pyton
"Is Surrogate Motherhood Moral?" *Humanist*, September 2001.

David Quinn
"Brave New World Rewound," *National Review*, July 13, 2001.

Lorilyn Rackl
"An Answer to Infertility Problems Raises Plenty of Questions," *Arlington Heights Daily Herald*, May 8, 2000.

William Reville
"No Need to Be Afraid of Genetic Engineering," *Irish Times* (Dublin), May 15, 2003.

Carol Sarler
"Trust the Science and Save a Child: Why Are Pro-lifers So Ready to Damn Something That Can Change for the Better the Lives of Millions?" *Observer*, December 16, 2001.

Cathy Sherry
"A Woman's Right, and Sometimes She's Not," *Sunday Age* (Melbourne), April 6, 2003.

William A. Silverman
"Unnatural Selection," *Pediatrics*, June 2001.

Rebecca L. Skloot
"Babies at Risk: Untested and Unregulated Procedures Are Used in U.S. Fertility Clinics," *Cleveland Plain Dealer*, February 26, 2003.

Christine Stolba
"Overcoming Motherhood: Pushing the Limits of Reproductive Choice," *Policy Review*, December 2002.

Jaylan S. Turkkan
"Why Cloning Makes Us So Uncomfortable," *Buffalo News*, January 12, 2003.

Nicholas Wade
"Clinics Hold More Embryos than Had Been Thought," *New York Times*, May 9, 2003.

Robert A. Weinberg
"The Cloning Clowns," *Prospect*, February 20, 2003.

Panayiotis Zavos
"Cloning Offers Chance for Infertile to Have Children," *Cincinnati Post*, August 15, 2001.

Index